T0227410

Social Work, Marriage, and Ethnicity

By looking at a variety of racial and ethnic groups in society, *Social Work, Marriage, and Ethnicity* examines the conventional knowledge, theories, and best practices relating to marriages. Contributors address marriage interventions, female empowerment, parenting, and cohabitation, as well as the variables which impact these situations, such as employment, housing, domestic violence, and HIV/AIDS, within appropriate and meaningful cultural contexts.

This book will be particularly useful for social workers working in many settings: clinical, community, research, policy implementation, faith-based, and other arenas that are available to couples in need of marital support. Marriage issues need to be addressed by social workers, given its status as a vital element in family strengthening and relationship stability. This book emboldens the case manager, community organizer, or immigration officer to address marital stresses and the demands faced by those couples most impacted by systemic inequality and barriers to cultural interventions.

This book was originally published as a special issue of the *Journal of Human Behavior in the Social Environment.*

Colita Nichols Fairfax is an Associate Professor, Honors College Liaison, and Nationally Certified Online Instructor in the Ethelyn R. Strong School of Social Work, Norfolk State University, Norfolk, Virginia, USA. Her major research interests include community theories, practice models, and policy analysis in areas of marriage, development, and mobilization strategies.

Social Work, Marriage, and Ethnicity

Policy and practice

Edited by
Colita Nichols Fairfax

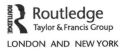

Routledge
Taylor & Francis Group

LONDON AND NEW YORK

First published 2016
by Routledge
2 Park Square, Milton Park, Abingdon, Oxon, OX14 4RN, UK

and by Routledge
711 Third Avenue, New York, NY 10017, USA

Routledge is an imprint of the Taylor & Francis Group, an informa business

British Library Cataloguing in Publication Data
A catalogue record for this book is available from the British Library

ISBN 13: 978-1-138-93217-3

Typeset in Times New Roman
by RefineCatch Limited, Bungay, Suffolk

Publisher's Note
The publisher accepts responsibility for any inconsistencies that may have
arisen during the conversion of this book from journal articles to book chapters,
namely the possible inclusion of journal terminology.

Disclaimer
Every effort has been made to contact copyright holders for their permission to
reprint material in this book. The publishers would be grateful to hear from any
copyright holder who is not here acknowledged and will undertake to rectify
any errors or omissions in future editions of this book.

Contents

Citation Information

The chapters in this book were originally published in the *Journal of Human Behavior in the Social Environment*, volume 24, issue 2 (February–March 2014). When citing this material, please use the original page numbering for each article, as follows:

For any permission-related enquiries please visit:
http://www.tandfonline.com/page/help/permissions

Notes on Contributors

Alean Al-Krenawi is former Dean and Professor at Memorial University's School of Social Work in Newfoundland, St. John's, Canada. He is former Chair of the Spitzer Department of Social Work at Ben-Gurion University of the Negev, Beer-Sheva, Israel.

Melissa Almenas is based at the Center for Safety and Change, New City, New York, USA.

Tricia Bent-Goodley is Professor of Social Work and Director of the Doctoral Program at Howard University School of Social Work, Washington DC, USA.

Giovani Burgos is Assistant Professor of Sociology at Stony Brook University, New York, USA.

Anthony De Jesús is Assistant Professor in the Department of Social Work and Latino Community Practice at the University of Saint Joseph, West Hartford, Connecticut, USA.

Pa Der Vang is Assistant Professor in the School of Social Work at St. Catherine University, St. Paul, Minnesota, USA.

Colita Nichols Fairfax is Associate Professor, Honors College Liaison, and Nationally Certified Online Instructor in the Ethelyn R. Strong School of Social Work, Norfolk State University, Norfolk, Virginia, USA.

Naomi Farber is Associate Professor in the College of Social Work at the University of South Carolina, Columbia, South Carolina, USA.

Pa Her is Assistant Professor in the Department of Social Science at New York City College of Technology, Brooklyn, New York, USA.

Magen Holgate is based in the School of Social Work at Brigham Young University, Provo, Utah, USA.

Kanata Jackson is Chair and Associate Professor in the Department of Management in the School of Business at Hampton University, Virginia, USA.

Stephen O. Jackson is based in the Department of Education at Memorial University of Newfoundland, St. John's, Canada.

Gordon E. Limb is Professor in the School of Social Work at Brigham Young University, Provo, Utah, USA.

Julie E. Miller-Cribbs is Professor and Director in the Anne and Henry Zarrow School of Social Work at the University of Oklahoma-Tulsa, Oklahoma, USA.

Peter Nguyen is Associate Professor in the School of Social Work at Virginia Commonwealth University, Richmond, Virginia, USA.

Noelle M. St. Vil is Assistant Professor of Social Work at Elizabethtown College, Elizabethtown, Pennsylvania, USA.

Jerilyn Tobler is based in the School of Social Work at Brigham Young University, Provo, Utah, USA.

William Velez is Professor in the Department of Sociology at the University of Wisconsin–Milwaukee, Milwaukee, USA.

Ingrid Phillips Whitaker is Associate Professor in the Department of Sociology and Criminal Justice at Old Dominion University, Norfolk, Virginia, USA.

Mark M. Whitaker is Associate Professor of Management in the School of Business at Hampton University, Virginia, USA.

Cindy White is based in the School of Social Work at Brigham Young University, Provo, Utah, USA.

Social Work, Marriage, and Ethnicity: Policy and Practice

Colita Nichols Fairfax

The Ethelyn R. Strong School of Social Work, Norfolk State University, Norfolk, Virginia, USA

This article provides a discussion about marriage with regard to social work policy and practice with cultural groups that experience life differently from predominantly White America. Marriage is influenced by culture, tradition, and economic reality supporting or hindering the success of marriages. Often, parenting is influenced by marriage, as roles are shared and meted through the resources provided by marriage. As an introduction, this article explains the unique contribution of each article in the special issue, showing the need for social work to respond more critically, urgently, and in threefold systemic fashion to create change in the lives of historically vulnerable populations in U.S. society.

INTRODUCTION

Contrary to various public opinions, marriage in America has become a public, politicized institution, entrenched in American societal structures, "in the Western model, people expect marriage to satisfy more of their psychological and social needs than ever before, free of the coercion, violence and gender inequalities that were tolerated in the past" (Coontz, 2005, p. 23). Policies have been passed about who can marry whom and what should occur within the confines of marriage. As a romanticized society, getting married is a major social benchmark, equally weighted with a college degree, military rank, and home ownership. However, if one is wealthy with adequate resources, marriage is easily eluded. Yet, for poor populations, particularly historically vulnerable racial and ethnic groups, the absence of marriage has had ramifications on resources, child rearing, relationships, social power, and family structure. Social workers trained in the academy evaluate the sustainability, virtue, and success of family life on the basis of the presence and endurance of long-lasting marriages. In fact, the mere absence of marriage stigmatizes families, subjecting divorced or never-married women as less virtuous if they are in need of relief and assistance.

The editor thanks Dr. Iris Carlton-Laney, professor of social work at the University of North Carolina, Chapel Hill, and Dr. Joyce O. Beckett, professor emerita of social work at Virginia Commonwealth University, for reviewing manuscripts and providing editorial guidance. The editor also thanks Dr. Marvin Feit, professor of social work at Norfolk State University, for suggesting a special issue about marriage.

Yet, as a profession, social work has not provided adequate scholarly practice and advocacy of serious labored thought of societal structures that sustain marriages, and ultimately poor family life, among economically vulnerable populations, from poor Whites to immigrants, from Native populations to Latinos. In fact, survey data among a sample ($N = 102$) of the BSW population at Norfolk State University, The Ethelyn R. Strong School of Social Work, 76 students answered no (77%), 22 students answered yes (22%), and 4 students answered that they didn't know (4%) to the question, "Do you think that social work generalist practice curriculum discuss marriage sufficiently?" This small sample reveals that among undergraduate social work students, marriage is a discerning subject in the proverbial human behavior and social environment curriculum. Scholarly attention to interpersonal aspects of marriage and direct practice responses (Beckett & Smith, 1981; Emery & White, 2006; Kissen, 2003; Pinderhughes, 2002) is also documented. Yet, the lack of national social work conference themes devoted to marriage issues and most vulnerable persons, lack of attention of think tanks, policy briefs, practice webinars, and the like indicates this neglect. The goal of this special issue, Social Work, Marriage, and Ethnicity, is to explore social work policy and practice solutions with people of color who are socially, economically, and politically vulnerable in American society. Perhaps a clarion call will sound to our profession, a vigorous and unapologetic challenge, and will elucidate the structural reasons for fragile families: "To be effective with low-income and minority populations, marriage programs must target the real-life challenges these couples face and not just relationship skills" (Bembry, 2011, p. 65).

A longitudinal case study of an African American married couple exemplifies the historic lack of systemic supports for the average couple of color. Curwood examined socioeconomic variables affecting middle-class couples between 1918 and 1942, uncovering a range of "very human problems of sexual conflict, precarious finances, and mental health" (2010, p. 158), showcasing traditionally that couples do not openly divulge and seek interventions. Due to stigma, shame, and the status of marriage in America, such private information is guarded, because other family members may be unduly impacted by these kinds of real social and mental health issues. The constant worry over money adds extreme stress. Since children are the pride of marriages, their well-being is of ultimate concern for couples struggling with fiscal, employment, and mental health issues. Curwood's longitudinal examination shows that social institutions have not been available to couples of color, and that married people are expected to conquer their affairs themselves. This has repercussions for social workers not only addressing marital issues but to advocate and implement marital intervention in all areas of public welfare, public education, employment sector, hospitals and medical centers, community, recreational, and private agencies and projects.

The remarkable national movement of marriage equality for the lesbian, gay, bisexual, transgender, and queer/questioning persons (LGBT-Q) community continues to gain momentum throughout each state, with states (Rhode Island, Vermont, Connecticut, Iowa, Massachusetts, Maine, New Hampshire, Vermont, Washington, certain jurisdictions of Maryland), and the District of Columbia passing marriage equality statutes for that community as of this writing. Blended or stepfamilies are growing, as many persons are marrying later in life (Chadiha, 1992). However, the national discussion about marriage among people of color remains dull and unattended. Even though the high-profile marriage of President Barack and Michelle Obama has created more conversations about marriage in the African American community (Chaney & Fairfax, 2012), social workers are absent in this dialogue with disadvantaged communities, where people of color struggle with scarce resources and opportunities. Opportunities that are systematically denied, due to recalcitrant economic and political behaviors that elude poor Whites and historical and contemporarily disadvantaged groups, are "results of entrapment in the societal projection process and having to live with constant conflict, confusion, and contradiction while trapped within a system that undermines functional roles" (Pinderhughes, 2002, p. 272). Community and clinical knowledge should incorporate direct practices with couples as well as parenting and socialization, gender-role behaviors and responsibilities, and economic sustainability. No serious analysis and strategies to combat marriage and community issues can be offered without social work intervention, given the intimate intersections of, and dimensions of our work with disadvantaged groups.

The dialogue remains truncated within a rigid and Eurocentric paradigm of marriage and the nuclear family, neglecting the resilience and value of extended family and community structures that are a very significant feature among people of color (Gerstel, 2011; Lundquist, 2004; Stack, 1974; Sudarkasa, 1996). Marriage is studied as an independent variable, without any historical and culturally relevant analysis of the role and endurance of marriages within an extended family structure. Community has also been studied as an isolated variable. Among people of color, extended family and community family (i.e., church family) are critical to philosophical ideas of how people understand themselves and their relationship to their environment. Those communities that are organized culturally and economically are able to enforce values and traditions that are meaningful. If a community is strong, its families are strong economically, culturally, and politically. If a community subsists as a weak and fragile entity, it stands to reason that families are fragile and cannot contribute economically and institutionally. Addressing family fragility means social workers must honestly advocate for institutional and economic changes in the structures of society (Johnson, Honnald, & Threlfall, 2011). St. Onge corroborates this view: "There is a direct relationship between the quality of life in a community and the capacity of its social institutions to address basic human needs, build community, promote social transformation, and achieve institutional change" (2013, p. 426). The articles in this issue will showcase the impact of community, family, and cultural traditions on human well-being, as many marriages are arranged and complementary to the historical traditions, as found with Eastern Indian couples (Regan, Lakhanpal, & Anguiano, 2012). However, the status of women in arranged marriages as complementary to economic and political independence that many women in America enjoy continues to be abated, as some of the contributions in this volume will discuss. Social workers must have this knowledge in order to practice successfully in these communities, where marriage and family life carry significant and traditional meaning, in areas of social and economic sustainability, which are not necessarily focused on total assimilation.

The George Bush Administration (2001–2009) provided millions of dollars to fund marriage promotion activities within public welfare through the Department of Health and Human Services-Administration for Children and Families (ACF). The primary goals were to fund healthy marriage and demonstration programs. Yet, even though the ACF has created healthy relationship initiatives, sponsored conferences, symposiums, faith-based projects and offered policy statements, it has not effectively engaged the business sector in blue-collar employment opportunities, human resource personnel to train and hire men of color, and aggressively engage in job coaching and professional skills of poor women. Funding through the ACF initiative also illuminated an agglomeration of research articulating the positive attributes of marriage, yet again, the structural reasons for low marriage rates, high divorce rates, and out-of-wedlock birthrates are minimized and ignored. We have not seen a shift of institutional systemic behavior toward people of color, nor has social work as a profession been involved in best practice outcomes. Researchers from other human science fields have been funded in positivist and practice research initiatives, without full participation from social work. This special issue hopes to engage social workers more and gain more attention from governmental entities to address marriage and community issues for sincere change in our society.

No serious scholar offers one antidote for any societal problem; marriage is not the antidote to the plethora of social illnesses that plague people of color and poor Whites. Yet, the omission of marriage practice and policy advocacy in our profession is ominous and elusive of serious change among the families and communities we serve. Nor would any discerning scholar suggest that every woman and man shall get married in their lifetime. What is offered in this special issue is the preponderance of evidence that shows that social work practice and policy analysis is vital in the marital and relationship education and intervention with people of color and economically vulnerable folk.

There are several societal entities sanctioning marriage as the preferred beginning of a family; ACF, religious organizations and denominations, political parties, and several social science disciplines have offered numerous studies to show the benefits of marriage as well. Yet these entities are unwilling to violate historic boundaries to convert recalcitrant structural advantages that one group of people have over others (Jimenez, 2009). Public law 104-199: The Defense of Marriage Act, enacted in 1996, denied federal recognition to same-sex couples, yet more poignantly, catapulted marriage as a public and political institution. However, poor marriages and poor people in general face significant hardships to maintain the bonds of marriage. So while marriage provides four conspicuous functions—"(1) it provides a source of intimate relationships; (2) it acts as a unit of economic cooperation and consumption; (3) it may produce and socialize children; and (4) it assigns social roles and status to individuals" (Strong, DeVault, & Cohen, 2008, p. 13)—research shows that cohabiting couples are providing some of the same functions, as cohabitation has become a vital stage in marriage formation (McGinnis, 2003).

There are decades of scientific studies to show the structural impact upon marriages among the poor. For example, there are observations that the drop in the marriage rate among disadvantaged groups is directly correlated with factors such as unemployment (Wilson, 1987, 1996), environmental realities of high crime, substance abuse (Western, 2004), health and mental health issues (Illovsky, 2003; Davis, 2011), younger generational ideas of female independence (Edin & Kefalas, 2005), and the health catastrophe of HIV/AIDS (Fullilove, 2006), revealing acerbic realities of marriage endurance when struggling without resources to sustain child development and ownership of homes and contribute to safe communities and follow healthy marriage patterns of public profiled and traditional couples. Social workers should not only have this knowledge but incorporate it within the engagement and knowledge acquisition phase of the client-worker pact.

The intersection of marriage in the many arenas social workers are employed is evident. Yet often marriage is conflated with a multitude of family issues. When we work with families intervening with the child welfare system, we are working with couples of the birth family and foster family (James & Wilson, 1991). Often our work with families strangled with a loved one with HIV/AIDS involves spouses. Edwards, Irving, and Hawkins report that "married women spent an absorbent amount of their time care-giving for their HIV positive husbands" (2011, p. 1368) and are often in need of social and emotional support. Our community practice work with homeless men, women, and children often requires us to discuss aspects of a relationship with an estranged spouse or the coping mechanisms that homeless couples use to endure such crisis.

Our work with women escaping violence requires introspective therapy with them about their marriage and needed skill sets for future healthy relationships. Bent-Goodley advises the following:

> As the field of social work moves forward, . . . there are five specific features or components of strategies [that] are critical in reducing intimate partner violence, and eliminating it in the lives of women and girls: (1) community and faith-based approaches, (2) healthy relationship education, (3) intersectional program strategies, (4) intergenerational approaches, and (5) culturally and developmentally proficient programs as part of solid practice. (2011, pp. 179–180)

Our work in eligibility should demand that not only we means-test for benefits but that we "mean well" for marital supports with impactful intervention. Those couples who are means-tested for eligibility are living in marginality, outside of substance, resources, money, and recognition, and are living within ambiguity (Holosko & Feit, 2004). Our work with ex-offenders requires relationship and marital intervention that parallels personal and parental development,

> because incarceration appears to undermine such high-quality relationships, low marriage rates among ex-offenders offers little support for the idea that women who have separated from men with criminal

records are necessarily at lower risk of violence, imprisonment may increase women's exposure to violence in the long run. (Western, 2004, p. 47)

Social workers can apply direct practice skills to assist military marriages to thrive in the midst of war and the transition from war. More evaluation is needed with American military families that show positive marital outcomes that are desired in civilian life, "event history models predicting the likelihood of marriage show that black civilians are less likely than white civilians to marry, whereas black and white military enlisters exhibit similar-and vary high-propensities to marry" (Lundquist, 2004, pp. 751–752). Paradoxically, the military environment is fraught with sexual violence and rape, robbing active-duty women who are married to civilians without legal protective guards that are often utilized in civilian life (Forgey & Badger, 2010).

Social workers should be completely involved in transition work with immigrant families, as America is turning brown. More evaluation is also needed with immigrant populations who are typically married and regulated through immigration law, which "permits government intervention at all points in a marriage [courtship stage, entry-wedding stage, intact marriage stage, exit stage], and even when a couple may divorce" (Abrams, 2007, p. 1628). Abrams's legal analysis is that immigration law privileges married couples with regard to obtaining immigrant visas and qualifying for an exception or waiver if there is ineligible denial entry or possible deportation. The implications for social workers are to create bridges of intervention and opportunities to meet the desires of populations in dialoguing about marriage and the possibility of tripartite interventions to meet social and economic needs of spouses.

SOCIAL WORK'S PROFESSIONAL RESPONSE

This special issue seeks to expand the boundaries of marriage dialogue in our profession. Although marriage is often conflated with family issues, marriage is not always specifically focused upon with the poor and people of color. As the devolution of government services continues, communities will require resourceful families to attenuate societal imbalances that permit suffering and violence that promote male/female unhealthiness, poor parenting, discontinued cultural traditions, fragile extended family life, financial suffering, and upward mobility. Yet resourceful families mean that marriages are healthy, culturally vibrant and nonviolent. Social workers should not abdicate such work to family science researchers, as our work is equally significant and necessary to stabilizing families and communities. The dichotomy between family researchers and social workers has not yielded better practice results, nor do we see a unified professional and academic voice that benefits those marriages, families, and communities that continue to be caricatured. Furthermore, the schism between government, industry, and the social sciences, including social work, fans the flames of social dissonance between impoverished and privileged groups, assuaging an accepted malaise in American society. Theories that will implement structural change resulting in economic advancement for people of color are quite relevant.

Theories not only guide our assumptions about families and society, they provide us with an interpretive lens for organizing observations and phenomena where the best helping practices applied. The contributors to this special issue articulate useful theories that underscore the social work response to marital phenomena. Theories that appear to be quite useful in articulating marital phenomena are found in family ecology theory, which emphasizes the influence of environmental factors upon families, as well as systems theory. For example, symbolic interaction theory helps us to evaluate the interactions that persons have with each other, which creates certain meanings that people use to behave in their relationships. Although it is completely appropriate in the vein of marriage education and healthy relationship education (Dion, 2005), this theory does not yield an analysis of how poor families of color interface with wider society to meet their resource needs independently and respectfully.

Another theoretical example is structural functionalism theory, which provides us with an interpretive framework of how families relate to society and how social workers would use appropriate skills to help families of color maximize their needs within a society that does not always value their historic and contemporary contributions as a group. This theory focuses upon how roles are implemented of family members with regard to family survival within American society. It provides us with how to engage best practices for families and communities roles that need support to advance socially.

Jerome Schiele has written about African-centered or Afrocentric theory in social work (2000), which utilizes the cultural traditions that African American families use to thrive, survive, and continue practices based in spirituality and the ritual of church attendance and involvement, extended family form, resource sharing, political advancement, generationally and community-influenced parenting of children, business ownership, and education attainment. It is a theory that also explains the human impact of living on the margin of American society based upon racial designation. Schiele explains centuries of racial and violent institutional behaviors and an unequal distribution of power and resources have produced a spiritual alienation, diminishing the quality of interpersonal and intergroup relations, with adverse social, psychological, and economic implications for people of African descent, and in fact, all groups of people in America (2000). The Afrocentric social work practitioner incorporates African philosophy, culture, and strategies tripartite to confront and engage in advancing poor families and communities who are ignored and neglected systemically based upon the racial structures that are inherent in American society.

Social workers must utilize theory to address policy outcomes that can significantly alter poverty and community distress. An example of a specific policy outcome at the state level may involve improving the economic conditions of low-income families through aggressive business engagement with local departments of social services, job coaching and training of high school students, apprenticing for high school seniors, and students at community colleges and for-profit educational institutions. Persons exiting prisons are vulnerable and shunned by family and community who are ashamed of them. They are homeless and are often exiled due to their inability to continue marriages and relationships that were shattered by their incarceration. They will benefit from economic training, as their families and communities will, particularly poor women who require financial independence.

IMPLICATIONS: WHAT SHOULD BE DONE?

The articles selected for this issue address many articulations and research about the role of marriage and the impact of community life among racial and ethnic groups in America. They reflect advancements in our knowledge of the effect of social policy in the lives of those who are an important part of the social fabric of American society. They confirm that social workers have a critical role to play in a meaningful national dialogue and best mezzo-practices about marriage and community life. The articles support a more active profession to articulate broadly approaches that allow for a marriage dialogue, without violating the self-determination value, a dearly held tenet. The evidence is clear that culturally based approaches yield better economic and social outcomes that social workers intervene with in all the arenas we labor in. A major consideration of public policy is that, given the push to legalize same-sex marriage from the LGBT-Q community, with all of the insurance and financial protections allowed, social workers should entertain more constructive dialogue with cohabitating couples, and non-married persons co-raising children that they do not have these considerations or protections. Even among extended families with resources, children born unto non-married parents may not receive insurance and fiduciary inheritances. Sharon Brown notes in her study that cohabitating is less financial stable and impacts psychological well-being and heightens depression of all involved (2000), as evidenced in her longitudinal study.

The articles expand the meaning of cultural competence. It is not simply acknowledging that there are racial differences but that there are significant lived experiences based upon race and ethnicity that should be included in every phase of the helping process with outcomes that are substantial to the lived economic and social realities of that cultural group. Whether Boricuas intermarry, as De Jesús and colleagues articulate, or whether teen female Hmong women choose to marry, as Pa Der Vang and Pa Her elucidate, these are issues that impact the quality of life of communities that are ignored and neglected. These studies show that mate choosing is an important cultural aspect of social mobility and self-esteem, and social workers should be poised to intervene with these pertinent choices with Puerto Rican, Hmong, and Vietnamese populations. In fact, the practice of narrative therapy, as suggested by Pa Der Vang and Pa Her, is applicable to personal self-esteem and self-understanding, as young women need interventions to organize and make sense of their cultural realities and their needs to embrace new ways of knowing who they are, toward achieving successful choices of careers and marriages, if they so choose. Cultural expectations among Vietnamese Americans, with responsibilities to families in both nations, have domestic violence and mental health stressors that render this community fragile, as discussed by Nguyen. Teaching unmarried parents to effectively work with each other to better parent their children is tantamount to child development, as articulated in this issue by Limb et al., Limb and Tobler, and Whitaker et al. Yet central to effective parenting is the model of healthy relationships that are culturally resolute. Bent-Goodley offers a culturally based intervention that seeks to fill a void in healthy relationship education, such as In-Circle, that responds to the realities of race and class within the African American community. Mezzo-practice intervention with couples must attend to building couple-knowledge of financial acumen, healthy lifestyle choices with regard to sexual and intimacy practices, medical practices and adherence, and couple-to-couple mentoring. In-Circle is an incredible intervention, as St. Vil reports in her article, balancing work and family impacts marital satisfaction among African Americans.

After 9/11, the Arab American community found itself victim of racial hatred and impiety. As a human-based science of helping and healing, social workers cannot succumb to bias and erroneous generalizations of an entire group of people in this new century. As Al-Krenawi and Jackson explore, traditions, marriage, and family are completely important to this population; thus, helping services must consider the values and traditions of Arab Americans when intervening with those who seek engagement. In this issue, Farber and Miller-Cribbs offer a compelling analysis with focused life histories, of face-to-face interviews with open-end questions, about marriage and relationship endurance of a sample population living within poverty that includes violence, abuse, and resource deprivation. This is human suffering of poor White women that remains neglected in popular culture, news, and social media, and is quite ignored among political powerbrokers and pundits. Social workers need to address practice interventions that attend the veracity of violence, poverty, and scarcity of resources rendering women powerless in resource attainment, and in building sustainable relationships with poor men who are bereft of relationship mentoring and skills coupled with economic security within interventions. Also added in this issue is the review of Congress and Gonzalez's edited book, reviewed by Sledge, which showcases the continued focus on social work's value of multicultural practice with families. Sledge found that specific practices with marriage is not as prevalent in multicultural practice as the contributors would prefer and as the studies show evidence for. This special journal issue provides a critical editorial comment, that empirical evidence is sorely needed to examine best practices for marriages among couples of color and the relationship between marriage and community sustainability.

Despite many caveats, social workers have a profound role to play in this public discourse, with appropriate practices and meaningful outcomes, as we are the first responders to family and community disintegration and devastation. The silence of the social work profession about the marriage crisis, coupled with cultural, community, and fiduciary aspects that add layers to the multi-problem phenomena we continue to experience in the field is poignant. Unless we equally address systemic and intimate interventions, we lose out on the potential to enact true change with couples of color, in this moment in time when sympathy toward these particular groups is absent among political powerbrokers and philanthropists. Our profession must work much more intricately with social services, community services boards, community outreach programs, and community practices to reevaluate and resuscitate our engagement and knowledge acquisition phase of intervention to include culturally relevant healthy relationship/marriage education possibilities. This kind of intervention bolsters confidence, self-esteem, and personal value of those who need to learn how to be in relationship with others and themselves. Our profession must work much more intricately with public policymakers to incorporate adequate funding for healthy relationship/marriage education in the traditional service markets and community practice environments. The evidence that this volume presents should push our profession to boldly address marriage and community for people of color and those vulnerable citizens who are a part of the fabric of American life, on the strengths of their cultural and lived realities.

REFERENCES

Abrams, K. (2007). Immigration law and the regulation of marriage. *Minnesota Law Review, 91*(56), 1626–1709.

Beckett, J. O., & Smith, A. D. (1981). Work and family roles: Egalitarian marriage in black and white families. *Social Service Review, 55*(2), 314–326.

Bembry, J. X. (2011). Strengthening fragile families through research and practice. *Journal of Family Social Work, 14*, 54–67.

Bent-Goodley, T. (2011). *The ultimate betrayal: A renewed look at intimate partner violence.* Washington, DC: NASW Press.

Brown, S. (2000). The effect of union type on psychological well-being: Depression among cohabitators versus marrieds. *Journal of Health and Social Behavior, 41*(3), 241–255.

Chadiha, L. (1992). Black husbands' economic problems and resiliency during the transition to marriage. *Families in Society, 73*(9), 542–552.

Chaney, C., & Fairfax, C. N. (2013). A change has come: The Obamas and the culture of Black marriage in America. *Ethnicities, 13*, 20–48.

Coontz, S. (2005). *Marriage, a history: From obedience to intimacy or how love conquered marriage.* New York, NY: Viking.

Curwood, A. C. (2010). *Stormy weather: Middle-class African American marriages between the two world wars.* Chapel Hill, NC: The University of North Carolina Press.

Davis, K, (2011), Involuntary commitment policy: Disparities in admissions of African American men to state mental hospitals. In J. H. Schiele (Ed.), *Social welfare policy: Regulation and resistance among people of color* (pp. 63–90). Thousand Oaks, CA: SAGE Publications,

Dion, M. B. (2005). Healthy marriage programs: Learning what works. *The Future of Children, 15*(2), 139–156.

Edin, K., & Kefalas, M. (2005). *Promises I can keep: Why poor women put motherhood before marriage.* Berkeley, CA: University of California Press.

Edwards, L. V., Irving, S. M,. & Hawkins, A. S. (2011). Till death do us part: Live experiences of HIV-positive married African American women. *The Qualitative Reports, 16*(5), 1361–1379. Retrieved from http://www.nova.edu/ssss/QR/QR16-5/edwards.pdf

Emery, P., & White, J. C. (2006). Clinical Issues with African-American and White women to marry in mid-life. *Clinical Social Work Journal, 34*(1), 23–44.

Forgey, M. A., & Badger, L. (2010). Patterns of intimate partner violence and associated risk factors among married enlisted female soldiers. *Violence and Victims, 25*(1), 45–61.

Fullilove, R. (2006). *African Americans, health disparities and HIV/AIDS: Recommendations for confronting the epidemic in Black America.* Washington, DC: The National Minority AIDS Council.

Gerstel, N. (2011). Rethinking families and community: The color, class, and centrality of extended kin ties. *Sociological Forum, 26*(1), 1–20.

Holosko, M. J., & Feit, M. D. (2005). Living in poverty in America today. *Journal of Health and Social Policy* (*now Social Work and Public Health*), *21*(1), 119–131.

Illovsky, M. (2003). *Mental health professionals, minorities and the poor*. New York, NY: Brunner-Routledge.

James, A. L., & Wilson, K. (1991). Marriage, social policy and social work. *Journal of Social Work Practice, 5*(2), 171–180.

Jimenez, J. (2009). *Social policy and social change: Toward the creation of social and economic justice*. Thousand Oaks, CA: SAGE.

Johnson, J. A., Honnold, J. A., & Threlfall, P. (2011). Impact of social capital on employment and marriage among low income single mothers. *Journal of Sociology and Social Welfare, 38*(4), 9–31.

Kissen, M. (2003). Why is marriage so difficult? A psychoanalyst's perspective. *Psychoanalytical Social Work, 10*(2), 5–19.

Lundquist, J. H. (2004). When race makes no difference: Marriage and the military. *Social Forces, 83*(2), 731–757.

McGinnis, S. (2003). Cohabitating, dating and the perceived costs of marriage: A model of marriage entry. *Journal of Marriage and Family, 65*(February), 105–116.

Pinderhughes, E. B. (2002). African American marriage in the 20th century. *Family Process, 41*(2), 269–282.

Regan, P. C., Lakhanpal, S., & Anguiano, C. (2012). Relationship outcomes in Indian-American love-based and arranged marriages. *Psychological Reports, 110*(3), 915–924.

Schiele, J. H. (2000). *Human services and the Afrocentric paradigm*. Binghamton, NY: Haworth Press.

Stack, C. B. (1974). *All our kin: Strategies for survival in a Black community*. New York: Harper & Row.

St. Onge, P. (2013). Cultural competency: Organizations and diverse populations. In M. E Weil, M. Reisch, & M. L. Ohmer (Eds.), *The handbook of community practice* (pp. 425–444), Thousand Oaks, CA: Sage.

Strong, B., DeVault, C., & Cohen T. F. (2008). *The marriage and family experience: Intimate relationships in a changing society* (10th ed.). Belmont, CA: Thomson Wadsworth.

Sudarkasa, N. (1996). *The strengths of our mothers: African and African American women and families: Essays and speeches*. Trenton, NJ: Africa World Press.

Western, B. (2004). *Incarceration, marriage and family life*. Princeton, NJ: Princeton University, Department of Sociology. Retrieved from https://www.russellsage.org/sites/all/files/u4/Western_Incarceration,%20Marriage,%20%26%20Family%20Life.pdf.

Wilson, W. J. (1987). *The truly disadvantaged*. Chicago, IL: University of Chicago Press.

Wilson, W. J. (1996). *When work disappears: The world of the new urban poor*. New York, NY: Albert Knopf.

Strengthening American Indian Couples' Relationship Quality to Improve Parenting

Gordon E. Limb, Cindy White, and Magen Holgate

School of Social Work, Brigham Young University, Provo, Utah, USA

Using Fragile Families data, this study examined the impact that relationship quality has on American Indian parenting and its consequences on children. Results indicated that the more support American Indian parents received from one another, the more positive interactions they had with their child. Additionally, while engagement increased and spanking decreased with more support received for unmarried American Indian mothers, support from the father impacted their engagement more so than those who were married. Therefore, implementation of culturally appropriate relationship enhancing and premarital programs could be beneficial to strengthening American Indian families and have a positive impact on parenting.

Recent social trends in broadening the definition of marriage and fertility have led to changes in family formation. Currently in the United States, 38.5% of children are born to unmarried couples, with significantly higher rates in populations of color (46.4%–69.3%; Hamilton, Ventura, Martin, & Sutton, 2005; Martin et al., 2011). Because of these trends, the Administration for Children and Families (ACF) Healthy Marriage Initiative began focusing on enhancement of relationship skills and union stability for couples. The purpose of this Initiative was to encourage couples to participate in premarital programs to help them acquire the knowledge and skills necessary to form and sustain a healthy marriage (ACF, 2010). Research has shown that participation in premarital intervention programs enhances many relationship aspects and reduces divorce rates (Fawcett, Hawkins, Blanchard, & Carroll, 2010; Stanley, Blumberg, & Markman, 1999).

While the impact of parenting and relationship quality of unmarried parents has been a concern generally, American Indian families are at even greater risk. For example, 52% of American Indian children lived in single-parent families in 2010 (Annie E. Casey Foundation, 2010). Few studies have examined specific parenting and relationship quality issues of American Indian couples. Therefore, the purpose of this study was to examine the impact that American Indian parents' relationship quality has on their parenting. The following section provides a brief synopsis of parenting and relationship quality issues generally, followed by specific attention given to how parenting and relationship quality issues impact American Indians.

PARENTING AND RELATIONSHIP QUALITY AMONG THE GENERAL POPULATION

Parenting can be stratified into positive behaviors—those that are beneficial to a child's development and include warmth, engagement, and responsiveness—and negative behaviors—those that can be detrimental to a child's development and include punitiveness, harshness, and hostility (Boyle et al., 2004; Collins, Maccoby, Steinberg, Hetherington, & Bornstein, 2000; Ho, Bluestein, & Jenkins, 2008). Parenting quality is impacted not only by positive and negative behaviors but also by factors such as a mother's physical and emotional health and stability. For example, cognitive-motivational competence and healthy socio-emotional development lead to attentive, warm, stimulating, and responsive caregiving (Belsky, Lerner, & Spanier, 1984; Cooper, Masi, & Vick, 2009; Margetts, 2005). Additionally, psychological maturity is correlated to parenting quality. Adolescent mothers exhibit greater risk for depression and parenting stress, which can diminish the mother's parenting effectiveness and interfere with the child's healthy development (Kalil, Ziol-Guest, & Coley, 2005).

Mothers are generally more involved than fathers in physically and psychologically caring for their children (Bianchi, Robinson, & Milkie, 2006; Nomaguchi & Milkie, 2003), but a young child's development is strongly influenced by interaction with both mother and father. Research also shows that the most significant predictors of a positive maternal attitude are a mother's satisfaction in the relationship with the birth father and his availability (Crnic, Greenberg, Robinson, & Ragozin, 2010), both strong indicators of overall relationship quality. Additionally, studies that focus on nonresident and divorced fathers have found that the quality of the parental relationship, regardless of marital status, is correlated to the father's frequency of visitation and financial support (Carlson & McLanahan, 2006; Harmon & Perry, 2011; Thompson & Laible, 1999).

In the general population, research suggests a positive correlation between the relationship quality of parents and their parenting behaviors (Carlson & McLanahan, 2006; Kitzmann, 2000; Krishnakumar & Buehler, 2000; Orbuch, Thornton, & Cancio, 2000). In many studies, relationship quality is measured on two levels: relationship conflict and relationship satisfaction (Kluwer & Johnson, 2007; Erel & Burman, 1995; Fincham, 1994).

Frequency of conflict is a common measure of relationship quality. Men and women typically respond differently to conflict and specifically on several key factors, including money, spending time together, sex, pregnancy, drug abuse, and partner faithfulness. In both married and unmarried populations, relationship satisfaction is significantly negatively correlated with conflict for both mothers and fathers (Cowan, Cowan, Shultz, & Hemming, 1994; Howes & Markman, 1989; Kluwer & Johnson, 2007). Additionally, unresolved interrelationship anger has been shown to have a negative impact on children. Of particular importance is the research showing the negative impacts of spanking (Carlson & McLanahan, 2006; Gershoff, 2002; Larzelere, Klein, Schumm, & Alibrando, 1989). When it is resolved, outcomes for children are more positive (Cummings, Ballard, El-Sheikh, & Lake, 1991; Moore, Kinghorn, & Bandy, 2011).

Factors contributing to relationship satisfaction include expressiveness, willingness to compromise, lack of criticism and insults, and encouragement of personal goals. Partner availability also enhances relationship satisfaction and can be measured by the level of physical and emotional support partners receive from one another. Supportiveness can include providing information and advice, help with routine tasks, assistance with child care, and financial support (Howard & Brooks-Gunn, 2009; Belksy, 1984).

In summary, the quality of the birth parents' relationship, including conflict and satisfaction, has a major impact on the mother's maternal attitude as well as to the father's paternal involvement and provision of financial support. Therefore, further examination of the correlation between relationship quality and parenting practices becomes integral to the strengthening of families, particularly unmarried American Indians.

PARENTING AND RELATIONSHIP QUALITY AMONG AMERICAN INDIANS

The out-of-wedlock birthrate for American Indian mothers in 2009 was 65%, yet few studies exist that examine relationships and parenting behaviors among American Indian couples (Martin et al., 2011). However, there is a federal program specifically created for marriage promotion among American Indians. As part of the ACF's implementation of the Healthy Marriage Initiative, the Native American Healthy Marriage Initiative was launched. This program was intended to strengthen couple relationships and families in American Indian communities through promoting healthy marriages, responsible fatherhood, and child well-being. It has specific focus on three elements: education and communication, the creation and enhancement of collaborations and partnerships, and identifying resources (Administration for American Indians, 2006). The impact of this program has yet to be determined, but the intent and scope of this program has widespread potential.

While empirical research dealing with relationship quality is limited, information about the dynamics of American Indian culture and families has been documented. Glover (2001) and Whitbeck (2006) both emphasize that the extended family, community, tribe, and clan are viewed as a collective piece of the family circle and often share parental responsibilities and roles with the birth parents. No distinction is made between blood relatives and those related by marriage, and all participate in the teaching, rearing, and passing along of cultural beliefs and traditions to the next generation (Limb, Hodge, & Panos, 2008). Caretaker roles in Native communities are much broader and involve many more people than non-Native communities.

Common values held by American Indian families include a deep and abiding respect for elders; making resources, such as housing, food, or transportation available to all within the extended family network; and an orientation toward what is best for the group rather than self-interest (Weaver & White, 1997). This notion of care within American Indian family systems includes not only providing for physical and emotional needs but also spiritual and cultural nurturing and mentoring as well (Besaw et al., 2004). Additionally, unlike Western conceptualization of family systems where as individuals become older they become more independent of their family of origin, in American Indian family systems, age and independence are negatively correlated. In other words, individuals assume greater kinship responsibilities as they grow older, and marriage does not simply unite two individuals but rather incorporates both into a larger kinship system (Red Horse, 1997).

While scholars who research American Indians often account for the traditional extended family structure and values, few studies have been conducted that examine contemporary urban American Indian couple relationships and parenting. Census data from the year 2010 indicate that 60% of American Indians now live in metropolitan rather than rural areas or on reservations (U. S. Department of Health and Human Services, 2011). Despite this movement from the reservations to urban centers, the value of extended relationships has remained intact (Lucero, 2007; Red Horse, 1997). Regardless of lifestyle patterns of nuclear families, extended family, including grandparents, aunts, and uncles, remains an integral part of child-rearing and familial responsibility (Red Horse, Lewis, Feit, & Decker, 1978). Therefore, the purpose of the current study was to examine the impact that American Indian parents' relationship quality has on their parenting. The goal is to contribute to the body of research on urban American Indian families by providing an in-depth examination of birth parents' relationship quality and the subsequent impact on their parenting behavior.

METHOD

Participants

This study uses data from the first two waves of the Fragile Families and Child Wellbeing study, a national, longitudinal study designed to examine the characteristics of unmarried parents, the relationships between mothers and the fathers, and the consequences for children (see Reichman, Teitler, Garfinkel, & McLanahan, 2001). The Fragile Families study follows a new birth cohort of approximately 4,900 children born between 1998 and 2000 (including 3,712 children born to unmarried parents and 1,186 children born to married parents) in 20 cities with populations over 200,000.

The Fragile Families study first interviewed mothers within 48 hours of birth while they were still in the hospital. Fathers were interviewed either in the hospital or wherever they could be located as soon as possible after the birth. Follow-up interviews were conducted at roughly 1 year and then every other year thereafter. For the current study, the sample was restricted to only those who self-identified as being American Indian. This yielded a total analysis sample of 222 American Indian mothers (comprising 4.5% of the total sample) and 144 American Indian fathers (comprising 3.8% of the total sample) from both waves. The Fragile Families data include several measures of relationship quality and parenting and are therefore well suited for examining the variables in this study (Carlson & McLanahan, 2006).

Measures

Parenting

Two measures of American Indian mothers' and fathers' parenting at the 1-year follow-up survey were examined as dependent variables. The first measure, engagement, was measured by mothers' and fathers' reports of the number of days in which they involved themselves in the following five activities with their child in the week before the interview: play imaginary games, sing songs or nursery rhymes, play inside with toys, read stories, and tell stories. Responses ranged from 0 to 7 days and were averaged to yield a composite measure of positive engagement ($\alpha = .926$).

The second measure assessed negative parenting behaviors and examined both mothers' and fathers' reports of the frequency that the child was spanked. Parents were asked whether they spanked the child in the month before the interview because she or he was misbehaving or acting up. Parents who replied affirmatively indicated whether spanking occurred "every day or nearly every day," "a few times a week," "a few times in the past month" or "only once or twice." Responses were coded into a five-scale variable, ranging from 1 (never) to 5 (every or nearly every day).

Parents' Relationship Quality

Two measures of parent's relationship quality were used as independent variables: support-iveness and frequency of conflict. The first measure, supportiveness, examined the mean scores across four items. These items assessed how often the other parent displayed the following four behaviors: (1) "Is fair and willing to compromise when you have a disagreement," (2) "Expresses affection or love for you," (3) "Insults or criticizes you or your ideas" (coding reversed), and (4) "Encourages or helps you to do things that are important to you." Responses ranged from 1 to 3 (1 = *never*, 2 = *sometimes*, and 3 = *often*) and were averaged to yield a composite score, with higher scores showing greater supportiveness ($\alpha = .996$).

Additionally, a measure of the change in supportiveness was also included in the current study. This measure was represented as the difference between an identical supportiveness measure at the baseline and 1-year follow-up surveys. A positive change score indicates that the relationship reportedly improved over time, and a negative score signifies a decrease over time.

The second measure, frequency of conflict, asked both parents during the baseline interview about the frequency of conflict on six topics: money, spending time together, sex, the pregnancy, drugs, and being faithful. Responses ranged from 1 to 3 (1 = *never*, 2 = *sometimes*, and 3 = *often*) and were averaged to yield a composite score, with higher scores showing more frequent conflict ($\alpha = .997$). The Fragile Families data did not allow for an examination of change on conflict over time because frequency of conflict was not measured at the 1-year follow-up survey.

Socio-Demographic Factors

Previous studies suggest a number of variables that could impact parents' relationship quality and parenting (see Carlson & McLanahan, 2006). For the current study, the following 13 socio-demographic variables at baseline were used to analyze parents' relationship quality and parenting. The age of each parent at the child's birth were designated as continuous variables. To represent family background, a dichotomy for whether each parent lived with both of his or her parents at age 15 was included.

Parent's economic conditions and current circumstances were measured by three variables: level of education, employment status, and household poverty status. Level of education was designated by four dummy variables: less than high school degree (reference category), high school degree, some college, and bachelor's degree or higher. Whether the father worked in the past week or the mother worked in the past year determined the parents' employment status. The household poverty status was measured by the household's income being divided by the federal poverty threshold in the baseline survey year (1998–2000). Three dummy variables were used to represent being poor (0–.99), near poor (1–2.49), and not poor (2.5 and higher).

Parents' physical health status ranged from 1 (*poor*) to 5 (*great*). Parents' substance abuse problems were calculated using a dummy variable, and responses were coded dichotomous as to whether the parents responded affirmatively that "drinking or drug use interfered with [their] work or personal relationships." The number of children in the household was a continuous variable. The frequency that each parent attended religious activities was measured using a Likert scale, ranging from 1 (*not at all*) to 5 (*once a week or more*). A dichotomous variable indicated whether the mother received prenatal care in the first trimester of her pregnancy. A dummy variable was created to represent whether the child was a boy. The parent reporting that their child had a difficult temperament was represented by the average of three items from the Emotionality, Activity, and Sociability Temperament Survey (Carlson & McLanahan, 2006). Finally, at the 1-year survey, mothers were asked how often their child fusses and cries, gets upset easily, and reacts very strongly when upset. The response choices ranged from 1 (*not at all like my child*) to 5 (*very much like my child*).

Data Analysis

The first set of analyses involved descriptive statistics to describe and compare relationship quality and parenting measures of married and unmarried couples at the time of the child's birth. For these analyses, both chi-square and *t*-tests were used to test differences in the two groups and were based on the normal approximation to the binomial distribution. Due to the exploratory nature of this study, a Bonferroni multiple-comparison test was not performed. The first set of analyses included socio-demographic variables that may be related to both relationship quality and parenting. Unless otherwise noted, the same measures were used for the mothers and fathers.

The second set of analyses involved linear regression models estimated to predict the two parenting measures (positive engagement and frequency of spanking) for mothers and fathers. Mothers and fathers were examined separately to better understand the different dynamics in how relationship quality affects parenting. Models for mothers and fathers were estimated together for each outcome using unrelated regressions that allowed the error terms to be correlated across mothers' and fathers' equations. For variables that were categorical or dichotomous, we used multinomial random assignment to fill in missing values where probabilities were determined by sample frequencies (Babbie, 2001; Raaijmakers, 1999).

RESULTS

When examining the socio-demographic factors of the mothers and fathers (Table 1), married and unmarried American Indian parents were similar on many items. However, married mothers were significantly older than unmarried mothers and, of married fathers, a significantly higher proportion (68.8%) lived with both of his parents at age 15 (compared to 50.9% of unmarried fathers). Only 20% of married mothers lived in poverty (compared to 40.7% of unmarried mothers), but a significantly higher proportion of married mothers reported being near poor (73.3% of married mothers were near poor compared to 41.8% of unmarried). Finally, a significantly higher proportion (88.9%) of married mothers noted that they received prenatal care in the first trimester of their pregnancy (compared to 74% of unmarried mothers).

Generally, American Indian parents reported having good to very good health. Relatively few American Indian parents reported substance abuse problems. Here, married mothers reported no substance abuse problems at all while 2.3% of unmarried mothers reported a problem. The mean number of children in each household was between one and two for both mothers and fathers.

TABLE 1
Descriptive Statistics by Marital Status at Baby's Birth

	Mother		*Father*	
Socio-Demographic Factors	*Unmarried*	*Married*	*Unmarried*	*Married*
Age at baby's birth (*M*, *SD*)	24.07 (5.99)	26.27 (5.12)*	26.17 (6.24)	25.91 (5.99)
Lived with both parents at age 15	55.9%	57.8%	50.9%	68.8%*
Focal child is first birth	41.2%	28.9%	40.2%	46.9%
Level of education				
Less than high school degree	69.5%	66.7%	37.3%	48.9%
High school degree	15.8%	15.6%	18.1%	15.6%
Some college	13%	13.3%	6.8%	4.4%
Bachelor's degree or higher	1.7%	4.4%	1.1%	2.2%
Worked in the last year or week	63.8%	53.3%	17.9%	18.8%
Household income-to-poverty ratio:				
Poor (0–.99)	40.7%	20%**	25.4%	33.3%
Near poor (1–2.49)	41.8%	73.3%**	32.2%	31.1%
Not poor (2.5+)	13.6%	15.6%	5.6%	6.7%
Health status (*M*, *SD*)	3.61 (.98)	3.36 (.71)	3.85 (.96)	3.88 (1.29)
Substance abuse problem	2.3%	0%	14.3%	12.5%
No. of children in household (*M*, *SD*)	1.31 (1.21)	1.58 (1.39)	1.74 (.74)	1.86 (.86)
Religious attendance (*M*, *SD*)	3.16 (1.37)	3.56 (.86)	2.88 (1.40)	2.56 (1.34)
Mother received prenatal care in 1st trimester	74%	88.9%*	NA	NA

*$p < 0.05$. **$p < 0.01$.

Married mothers reported more religious attendance than those mothers who were not married. This was not true for unmarried fathers, as they reported more religious attendance than their married counterparts. It is important to note that due to the lack of specificity within the questions on this variable, we were not able to determine whether religious attendance included a cultural focus or participating in a Native American church.

Table 2 provides the relationship quality and parenting measures reported by married and unmarried American Indian parents. Although there were no significant differences between married and unmarried American Indian parents in overall supportiveness, engagement, and conflict, there was significant difference for engagement between married and unmarried fathers. Here, American Indian fathers who were not married responded that they were more engaged with their children at the 1-year follow-up survey (4.65 compared to 4.12, respectively). On the other hand, American Indian mothers' engagement was higher for those who were married.

Regression Analyses

Results from the linear regression predicting American Indian parenting are reported in Table 3. For both mothers and fathers, the level of supportiveness in the parents' relationship at the child's birth and at the 1-year follow-up was positively associated with parent-child engagement, with the mothers being statistically significant. Good health status was positively and statistically significantly associated with positive engagement for mothers. Also, the worse American Indian fathers fared in health status, the more likely they were to spank their child. This finding was significant.

For American Indian mothers, there was no significant association between religious attendance and parenting. However, religious attendance for American Indian fathers was significantly and negatively correlated on engagement with their child. Not being poor was positively and significantly associated with mother engagement, and having a child with a difficult temperament was significantly and negatively correlated to a decrease in mothers' engagement with the child.

Table 4 contains information on differences in relationship quality as related to parenting between married and unmarried American Indian couples. Among the fathers, there were no statistically significant interaction differences between unmarried and married. Thus, the association between couple relationship quality and parenting appears to be similar for both unmarried fathers

TABLE 2
Relationship Quality and Parenting Measures Reported by Married and
Unmarried American Indian Parents

Measure	Married M (SD)	Unmarried M (SD)
Parents' relationship quality		
Supportiveness at time of birth	2.66 (.122)	2.66 (.236)
Change in supportiveness, birth to 1 year	0.08 (.242)	0.09 (.263)
Frequency of conflict at time of birth	1.41 (.142)	1.42 (.217)
Mother's parenting at 1 year		
Engagement	5.10 (1.03)	4.86 (1.06)
Frequency of spanking	1.18 (.650)	1.18 (.501)
Father's parenting at 1 year		
Engagement	4.12 (1.12)	4.65 (1.15)*
Frequency of spanking	2.64 (1.77)	2.68 (.391)
N	45	177

*$p < 0.05$.

TABLE 3
Results from Linear Regression Predicting American Indian Parenting Behaviors

| | Mothers Parenting | | Fathers Parenting | |
| | Engagement Coefficient (SE) | Spanking Coefficient (SE) | Engagement Coefficient (SE) | Spanking Coefficient (SE) |
Measure				
Parents relationship quality (mother-father average)				
Supportiveness	.153 (.40)*	−.107 (.19)	.039 (.45)	.050 (.14)
Change in supportiveness	.013 (.34)	−.083 (.16)	.049 (.38)	.151 (.11)*
Frequency of conflict	−.107 (.43)	−.036 (.20)	−.008 (.48)	−.019 (.15)
Socio-demographic variables				
Age at baby's birth	.109 (.01)	−.085 (.01)	.084 (.02)	−.003 (.01)
Parent lived with both parents at age 15	−.018 (.14)	−.043 (.07)	.020 (.20)	.013 (.06)
Focal child is first birth	.000 (.15)	.009 (.07)	−.105 (.20)	−.053 (.06)
Worked in the last year/week	.039 (.15)	.075 (.07)	.022 (.25)	.102 (.08)
Health status	.207 (.07)**	.087 (.04)	.080 (.10)	−.231 (.03)**
Substance abuse problem	.021 (.54)	.018 (.27)	−.050 (.28)	−.019 (.09)
Number of children in household	.030 (.06)	−.032 (.03)	−.050 (.13)	−.049 (.04)
Religious attendance	−.019 (.05)	−.003 (.03)	−.246 (.07)**	−.090 (.02)
Child is a boy	−.047 (.14)	.037 (.07)	−.049 (.20)	−.065 (.06)
Mother received prenatal care in 1st trimester	.136 (.17)*	−.057 (.09)	NA	NA
Level of education				
Less than high school degree	−.113 (.15)	−.065 (.08)	−.113 (.20)	.013 (.06)
High school degree	.040 (.20)	.063 (.10)	.018 (.22)	.044 (.07)
Some college	.079 (.21)	.045 (.11)	.107 (.33)	−.088 (.10)
Bachelor's degree or higher	.075 (.48)	−.051 (.24)	.106 (.68)	.000 (.21)
Household income-to-poverty ratio				
Poor (0–.99)	.097 (.15)	.130 (.07)	.123 (.20)	.066 (.06)
Near poor (1–2.49)	−.213 (.14)	−.106 (.07)	−.135 (.19)	−.118 (.06)
Not poor (2.5+)	.154 (.20)*	−.088 (.10)	.025 (.34)	.091 (.10)
Child has difficult temperament	−.205 (.07)**	−.135 (.03)	−.001 (.09)	−.113 (.03)

*$p < 0.05$. **$p < 0.01$.

and married American Indian fathers across most measures examined for this set of analyses. For the full sample of American Indian mothers, supportiveness in the parental relationship had a positive and significant interaction with engagement. The same was found for the unmarried sample. The last set of analyses explored the interaction between relationship quality and parenting for unmarried American Indian couples based on whether the child was the first born. The data showed that mothers who were not married and were first-time mothers significantly improved their engagement when they had more support from the baby's father.

DISCUSSION

Very little is known regarding the correlation between American Indian couple relationship quality and parenting. This study was designed to address this gap in the literature. Therefore, the purpose of this study was to examine the impact that American Indian parent's relationship quality had on their parenting. As a result, three overall patterns of findings were identified. The first overall

TABLE 4
Results from Linear Regression Predicting Married and Unmarried American Indian Parent's Engagement and Spanking

Measure	Engagement Coefficient (SE)	Spanking Coefficient (SE)
Marital status (full sample)		
Mothers parenting:		
Supportiveness	.190 (.24)**	−.103 (.12)
Change in supportiveness	−.035 (.20)	−.054 (.10)
Conflict	−.024 (.25)	.042 (.13)
Married × supportiveness	.088 (.50)	−.263 (.31)
Married × change in supportiveness	−.088 (.50)	.263 (.31)
Married × conflict	NA	NA
Father's parenting:		
Supportiveness	.031 (.33)	−.073 (.10)
Change in supportiveness	.049 (.25)	.063 (.08)
Conflict	.001 (.32)	.008 (.10)
Married × supportiveness	−.159 (.54)	−.047 (.09)
Married × change in supportiveness	.188 (.50)	−.016 (.08)
Married × conflict	.064 (.72)	−.024 (.11)
Unmarried sample		
Mother's parenting:		
Supportiveness	.211 (.28)**	−.047 (.13)
Change in supportiveness	−.017 (.22)	−.143 (.10)
Conflict	−.026 (.25)	.050 (.12)
Father's parenting:		
Supportiveness	.090 (.41)	−.089 (.14)
Change in supportiveness	.017 (.28)	.076 (.09)
Conflict	−.024 (.35)	.010 (.12)
First birth vs. later birth (unmarried sample)		
Mother's parenting:		
First birth × supportiveness	.289 (.39)*	.011 (.19)
First birth × change in supportiveness	−.149 (.32)	−.181 (.14)
First birth × conflict	−.016 (.44)	.101 (.20)
Father's parenting:		
First birth × supportiveness	.122 (.70)	.234 (.11)
First birth × change in supportiveness	−.057 (.46)	−.243 (.07)
First birth × conflict	−.008 (.51)	−.037 (.08)

*$p < 0.05$. **$p < 0.01$.

pattern indicated that the more support American Indian parents received from one another, the more they had positive interaction with their child. Increased support between partners also appeared to reduce the overall rate that American Indian parents spanked their child.

Together, these findings suggest that supportive relationships between American Indian mothers and fathers are important for positive parenting of very young children. Similar findings were also noted in previous research done by Carlson and McLanahan (2006) with the full Fragile Families sample as well as other scholars regarding positive spillover in married and unmarried relationships to parenting (e.g., Cox, Owen, Lewis, & Henderson, 1989; Krishnakumar & Buehler, 2000; McLanahan & Beck, 2010). The second pattern of results dealt with how marital status related to relationship quality and parenting. Here, results showed that for American Indian mothers, being married was associated with greater engagement with their child. For American Indian fathers, this was not the case, as unmarried fathers were more engaged with their children than those who were married. While this might imply advocating for fathers not to be married, one possible explanation for this finding could be cultural. Whether married or unmarried, American Indian fathers are still part of the community system to engage and care for the child. While further research is needed to flush this out in urban families, the American Indian father-child relationship does appear to have some unique cultural features.

Overall, this study found that marriage was positively associated with a variety of protective factors for American Indians including parents being older, more family involvement, greater financial stability, less substance abuse, and more prenatal care. These factors appear to be similar for the total sample population regardless of race. In the general sample, prior research reported married parents were much more likely than unmarried parents to have graduated from college, be financially stable, attend religious services more frequently, and receive prenatal care; whereas unmarried parents were more likely to have a child with a difficult temperament (Carlson & McLanahan, 2006). The promotion of marriage among American Indians is still appropriate for parenting, but it appears to be even more positive for mother's engagement with their child. Again, further research is needed to shed light on this topic.

Finally, the association between couple relationship quality and parenting appears to be similar for both unmarried and married American Indian fathers. Here, incorporating a collectivistic cultural expectation that is present in many Native communities, one might expect the father, regardless of whether he is married or is not, to be involved with his children. Further, while the father and mother may not be together, extended family would still play an important role in this relationship and would be actively involved with the children.

The third pattern of results suggests that while engagement increased and spanking decreased with more support received generally, for American Indian mothers who were not married, support from the father impacted their engagement more than those who were married. For those who were married, supportiveness in the relationship correlated to decreased spanking more so than for unmarried mothers. It may be that strengthening couple relationships among American Indian mothers and fathers may result in unmarried mothers being more positively engaged with their children and married mothers spanking their children less. This finding mirrors what Carlson and McLanahan (2006) found and further suggests that the strengthening of parental relationships can result in better parenting in American Indian mothers and fathers.

Finally, findings revealed that a number of socio-demographic factors impact American Indian parenting and the parental relationship. Higher engagement was associated with being older, more educated, and good health status. It is also important to note that the quality of the parental relationship was just as important for parents who had already had a child as it was for parents for whom the child was their first. Further, as noted earlier, American Indian parents who were married tended to be more financially stable, less susceptible to substance abuse, and more likely to have received prenatal care in the first trimester. As a result, we found that marriage was positively associated with many protective factors examined in this study.

This study has several limitations to take into consideration. First, the American Indian sample size was somewhat small. In analyzing a smaller sample size, power issues make it difficult to find statistically significant results. Second, we recognize that the use of self-report data and selecting variables from the 1-year follow-up and other variables from the baseline year could lead to response bias. Third, our study included American Indian mothers and fathers, but not all of their partners were American Indian. Hence, the results of our study may have had different outcomes had we limited our study to only include American Indian mothers who had children with American Indian fathers and vice versa. Fourth, this study utilized respondents who lived in large urban areas and oversampled for unmarried parents. Had the respondents been from rural or reservation areas or a different relationship our findings may have been different. Taking location, sample size, and sample selection factors into account, our findings regarding how American Indian parents' relationship quality affects their parenting may be limited and cannot be generalized to all American Indian parents.

Implications

Findings from this study suggest that implementation of premarital or relationship enhancing programs for clinicians working with American Indian couples, regardless of whether they are married or unmarried, may be beneficial to increasing stability and strengthening American Indian families. Here, research suggests that well-designed premarital and postmarital intervention programs can strengthen couple relationships, enhance marital stability, and reduce relationship stress (Fawcett et al., 2010; McLanahan & Beck, 2010; Stanley, 2001). Fawcett et al. suggest the need for marital intervention programs that emphasize commitment, sacrifice, and forgiveness and the skills that promote marital quality such as generosity, goodwill, other-centeredness, and self-control (p. 236). Intervention programs that utilize elements of cognitive-behavioral theory have also been found to be effective in reducing relationship stress (Epstein & Baucom, 2002).

Clinicians can also use intervention programs, implemented during specific transition times (such as marriage, parenthood, and divorces) to strengthen a number of relationship quality issues (McLanahan & Beck, 2010). For example, programs like The Prevention and Relationship Enhancement Program and Becoming a Family Program have been found to be effective in improving communication skill among engaged couples as they negotiated parenthood transitions (Cowan et al., 1985; Dion, 2005). These can include modification of unrealistic expectations, correction of faulty attributions, and the use of self-instructional procedures to decrease destructive interactions (Epstein, 1982). Similarly, the Native American Healthy Marriage Initiative offers resources and trainings to help American Indian couples and families. As a result, a number of empirically validated relationship enhancement programs are available to clinicians to use with their clients. Also, utilizing a community-based strategy that includes involvement and support of the extended family has been found to be effective in helping couple relationship enhancement and parenting (Laurenceau, Stanley, Olmos-Gallo, Baucom, & Markman, 2004).

While few of these have been tested with American Indians, preliminary findings suggest that American Indian couples are similar to the general population in many areas and would benefit from many of these intervention programs. However, prior research and findings from this study would suggest two cultural elements for clinicians to consider when working with American Indian couples. First, as noted earlier, it is important to involve extended family as clinicians provide services to strengthen relationship quality and parenting. Second, there appear to be cultural factors associated with American Indian father-child engagement. It is important for clinicians to be aware of this unique aspect as they provide services to fathers and their children.

Conclusion

With out-of-wedlock birth rates on the rise, especially among populations of color, it is important to recognize the impact this has on children. Within the United States, more than one in tthree children are born to unmarried couples (Hamilton et al., 2005). This study is a first for investigating how the quality of the relationship of American Indian parents affects the parenting their children receive. While research suggests that for the general population, as parental relationships improve so does their parenting (see Carlson & McLanahan, 2006; McLanahan & Beck, 2010), we found that this was also true for American Indian parents, regardless of their marital status. Therefore, strengthening not only married but also unmarried couple relationships could enhance the parenting American Indian children receive. For those working with the American Indian population, implementation of culturally appropriate premarital or relationship enhancing programs, including involvement in the Native American Healthy Marriage Initiative, may prove beneficial to increasing stability and strengthening American Indian families.

REFERENCES

Administration for American Indians. (2006). *National healthy marriage resource center: Fast facts.* Washington, DC: Administration for Children and Families.

Administration for Children and Families, U.S. Department of Health and Human Services. (2010). Healthy Marriage Initiative. Retrieved from http://www.acf.hhs.gov/healthymarriage/

Annie E. Casey Foundation. (2010). Children in single-parent families by race. Retrieved from http://datacenter.kidscount. org/data/tables/107-children-in-single-parent-families-by#detailed/1/any/false/867,133,38,35,18/10,168,9,12,1,13, 185/432,431

Babbie, E. (2001). *The practice of social research* (9th ed.). Belmont, CA: Wadsworth/Thomson.

Belsky, J., Lerner, R. M., & Spanier, G. B. (1984). *The child in the family.* Reading, MA: Addison-Wesley.

Besaw, A., Kalt, J. P., Lee, A., Sethi, J., Wilson, J. B., & Zemler, M. (2004). The context and meaning of family strengthening in Indian America. A Report to the Annie A. Casey Foundation by the Harvard Project on American Indian Economic Development. Retrieved at http://www.aecf.org/upload/PublicationFiles/fs_indian_america.pdf.

Bianchi, S. M., Robinson, J. P., & Milkie, M. A. (2006). *Changing rhythms of American family life.* New York, NY: Sage.

Boyle, M. H., Jenkins, J. M., Katholiki, G., Cairney, J., Duku, E., & Racine, Y. (2004). Differential-maternal parenting behavior: Estimating within- and between-family effects on children. *Child Development, 75*(5), 1457–1476.

Carlson, M. J., & McLanahan, S. S. (2006). Strengthening unmarried families: Could enhancing couple relationships also improve parenting? *Social Service Review, 80*(2), 297–321.

Collins, W. A., Maccoby, E. E., Steinberg, L., Hetherington, E. M., & Bornstein, J. II. (2000). Contemporary research on parenting: The case for nature and nurture. *American Psychologist, 55*(2), 218–232.

Cooper, J. L., Masi, R., & Vick, J. (2009). Social-emotional development in early childhood. National Center for Children in Poverty Brief. Retrieved from http://www.nccp.org/publications/pdf/text_882.pdf

Cowan, C. P., Cowan, P. A., Heming, G., Garrett, E., Coysh, W. S., Curtis-Boles, H., & Boles III, A. J. (1985). Transitions to parenthood: His, hers, and theirs. *Journal of Family Issues, 6*(4), 451–481.

Cowan, P. A., Cowan, C. P., Schulz, M. S., & Heming, G. (1994). Prebirth to preschool family factors in children's adaptation to kindergarten. In R. D. Parke and S. G. Kellam (Eds.), *Exploring family relationships with other social contexts* (pp. 75–114). Hillsdale, NJ: Erlbaum.

Cox, M. J., Owen, M. R., Lewis, J. M., & Henderson, V. K. (1989). Marriage, adult adjustment, and early parenting. *Child Development, 60*(5), 1015–1024.

Crnic K. A., Greenberg, M. T., Robinson, N. M., & Ragozin, A. S. (2010). Maternal stress and social support: Effects on the mother-infant relationship from birth to eighteen months. *American Journal of Orthopsychiatry, 54*(2), 224–235.

Cummings, E., Ballard, M., El-Sheikh, M., & Lake, M. (1991). Resolution and children's responses to interadult anger. *Developmental Psychology, 27*(3), 462–470.

Dion, M. R. (2005). Healthy marriage programs: Learning what works. *Future of Children, 15*(2), 139–156.

Epstein, N. (1982). Cognitive therapy with couples. *The American Journal of Family Therapy, 10*(1), 5–16.

Epstein, N. B., & Baucom, D. H. (2002). *Enhanced cognitive-behavioral therapy for couples: A contextual approach.* Washington, DC: American Psychological Association.

Erel, O., & Burman, B. (1995). Interrelatedness of marital relations and parent-child relations: A meta-analytic review. *Psychological Bulletin, 118*(1), 108–132.

Fawcett, E. B., Hawkins, A. J., Blanchard, V. L., & Carroll, J. S. (2010). Do premarital education programs really work? A meta-analytic study. *Family Relations, 59*(3), 232–239.

Fincham, F. D. (1994). Understanding the association between marital conflict and child adjustment: An overview. *Journal of Social and Personal Relationships, 14*(3), 357–372.

Gershoff, E. T. (2002). Corporal punishment by parents and associated child behaviors and experiences: A meta-analytic and theoretical review. *Psychological Bulletin, 128*(4), 539–579.

Glover, G. (2001). Parenting in Native American families. In N. B. Webb (Ed.), *Culturally diverse parent-child and family relationships: A guide for social workers and other practitioners* (pp. 205–231). New York, NY: Columbia University Press.

Hamilton, B. E., Ventura, S. J., Martin, J. A., &. Sutton, P. D. (2005). *Preliminary births for 2004. Health E-Stats.* Hyattsville, MD: U. S. Department of Health and Human Services, Center for Disease Control and Prevention, National Center for Health Statistics.

Harmon, D. K., & Perry, A. R. (2011). Fathers' unaccounted contributions: Paternal involvement and maternal stress. *Families in Society, 92*(2), 176–182.

Ho, C., Bluestein, D. N., & Jenkins, J. M. (2008). Cultural differences in the relationship between parenting and children's behavior. *Developmental Psychology, 44*(2), 507–522.

Howard, K. S., & Brooks-Gunn, J. (2009). Relationship supportiveness during the transition to parenting among married and unmarried parents. *Parenting: Science and Practice, 9,* 123–142.

Howes, P., & Markman, H. J. (1989). Marital quality and child functioning: A longitudinal investigation. *Child Development, 60,* 1044–1051.

Kalil, A., Ziol-Guest, K. M., & Coley, R. L. (2005). Perception of father involvement patterns in teenage-mother families: Predictors and links to mother's psychological adjustment. *Family Relations, 54*(2), 197–211.

Kitzmann, K. M. (2000). Effects of marital conflict on subsequent triadic family interactions and parenting. *Developmental Psychology, 36*(1), 3–13.

Kluwer, E. S., & Johnson, M. D. (2007). Conflict frequency and relationship quality across the transition to parenthood. *Journal of Marriage and Family, 69*(5), 1089–1106.

Krishnakumar, A., & Buehler, C. (2000). Interparental conflict and parenting practices: A meta-analysis. *Family Relations, 49*(1), 25–44.

Larzelere, R. E., Klein, M., Schumm, W. R., & Alibrando, S. A. (1989). Relations of spanking and other parenting characteristics to self-esteem and perceived fairness of parental discipline. *Psychological Reports, 64,* 1140–1142.

Laurenceau, J. P., Stanley, S. M., Olmos-Gallo, A., Baucom, B., & Markman, H. J. (2004). Community-based prevention of marital dysfunction: Multilevel modeling of a randomized effectiveness study. *Journal of Consulting and Clinical Psychology, 72*(6), 933–943.

Limb, G., Hodge, D., & Panos, P. (2008). Understanding the relational world view in Indian families. *Journal of Public Child Welfare, 2*(3), 383–397.

Lucero, N. M. (2007). Working with urban American Indian families with child protection and substance abuse challenges. Retrieved from http://www.americanhumane.org/assets/pdfs/children/pc-rmqic-dif-guide.pdf

Margetts, K. (2005). Responsive caregiving: Reducing the stress in infant toddler care. *International Journal of Early Childhood, 37*(2), 77–84.

Martin, J. A., Hamilton, B. E., Ventura, S. J., Osterman, M., Kirmeyer, S., Mathews, T., . . . Wilson, E. C. (2011). National Vital Statistics Reports. Births: Final data for 2009. Retrieved from http://www.cdc.agov/nchs/data/nvsr/nvsr60/nvsr60_01.pdf

McLanahan, S., & Beck, A. (2010). Parental relationships in fragile families. *The Future of Children, 20*(2), 17–37.

Moore, K. A., Kinghorn, A., & Bandy, T. (2011). Parental relationship quality and child outcomes across subgroups. Child Trends Research Brief. Retrieved from http://www.childtrends.org/Files/Child_Trends-2011_04_04_RB_Marital Happiness.pdf

Nomaguchi, K., & Milkie, M. (2003). Costs and rewards of children: The effects of becoming a parent on adults' lives. *Journal of Marriage and Family, 65*(2), 356–374.

Orbuch, T. L., Thornton, A., & Cancio, J. (2000). The impact of marital quality, divorce, and remarriage on the relationships between parents and their children. *Marriage and Family Review, 29*(4), 221–246.

Raaijmakers, Q. A. (1999). Effectiveness of different missing data treatments in surveys with likert-type data: Introducing the relative mean substitution approach. *Educational and Psychological Measurements, 59,* 725–748.

Red Horse, J. (1997). Traditional American Indian family systems. *Family Systems & Health, 15,* 243–250.

Red Horse, J., Lewis, R., Feit, M., & Decker, J. (1978). Family behaviors of urban American Indians. *Social Casework, 59,* 67–72.

Reichman, N. E., Teitler, J. O., Garfinkel, I., & McLanahan, S. S. (2001). Fragile families: Sample and design. *Children and Youth Services Review, 23*(4/5), 303–326.

Stanley, S. M. (2001). Making a case for premarital education. *Family Relations, 50*(3), 272–280.

Stanley, S. M., Blumberg, S. L., & Markman., H. J. (1999). Helping couples fight for their marriages. In R. Berger & M. T. Hannah (Eds.), *Preventive approaches in couples therapy* (pp. 279–303). New York, NY: Brunner/Mazel.

Thompson, R. A., & Laible, D. J. (1999). Noncustodial parents. In M. E. Lamb (Ed.), *Parenting and child development in "nontraditional" families* (pp. 103–123). Mahwah, NJ: Erlbaum.

U.S. Department of Health and Human Services. (2011). American Indian/Alaska Native profile. Retrieved from http://minorityhealth.hhs.gov/templates/browse.aspx?lvl=2&lvlID=52

Whitbeck, L. B. (2006). Some guiding assumptions and a theoretical model for developing culturally specific preventions with Native American people. *Journal of Community Psychology, 34*(2), 183–192.

White, L. (1999). Contagion in family affection: Mothers, fathers, and young adult children. *Journal of Marriage and the Family, 61*(2), 284–294.

Weaver, H., & White, B. (1997). The Native American family circle: Roots of resiliency. *Journal of Family Social Work, 2*(1), 67–79.

In Circle: A Healthy Relationship, Domestic Violence, and HIV Intervention for African American Couples

Tricia Bent-Goodley

School of Social Work, Howard University, Washington, DC, USA

While marriage and healthy relationship education has grown, limited interventions have been developed specifically to support the development and flourishing of African American couples. African Americans are also disproportionately impacted by HIV/AIDS and are more likely to experience lethality and serious injury due to domestic violence compared to Whites. Despite this, African American couples have been resilient and managed to thrive in relationships. Little has been done to capture these strategies, build on cultural strengths, and design an intervention specifically crafted for this population. This article describes an intervention "In Circle" developed, implemented, and evaluated for African American couples to support healthy relationship and healthy marriage education. The intervention is based on an Ancient Egyptian value system and undergirded by three integrated theoretical perspectives. The article also includes implications for practice and research.

Marriage statistics in the black community are often viewed as disparaging. Between 1950 and 1996, the rate of Black marriage fell from 78% to 34% (Blackman, Clayton, Glenn, Malone-Colon, & Roberts, 2005). Black couples also have an increased chance of experiencing divorce primarily due to severe stressors associated with unemployment, poverty, and economic stressors (O'Connor, 2006). Yet, African Americans still have a desire to get married. In fact, 77% of Blacks compared to 83% of Whites have a desire to be married, despite the fact that the rewards of marriage are often not discussed (Blackman et al., 2005). Black married couples enjoy a higher income, a reduced likelihood to live in poverty, increased happiness, and improved health outcomes, particularly for African American males (Bent-Goodley, in press).

Despite the above, little has been done to offer healthy relationship education to Black couples. It is often assumed that individuals learn what it means to be in a healthy relationship. Yet, not only has it been found that individuals are often not socialized into what it means to be in a healthy relationship, but they often do not have a model of what that relationship looks like (Bent-Goodley & Williams, 2008). Consequently, individuals base their relationship skills on what they have seen from others and on television, which can lead to problems in the relationship. The declining number of fathers in the Black home also impacts men having less socialization around what it means to be in a healthy relationship. For those healthy relationship education curricula, there are few developed that are philosophically and conceptually rooted and designed for this population (Blackman et al., 2005). Having an intervention that is uniquely created for African Americans allows one to structure a dialogue that is centered in the experience of the population from the values driving the program to the materials and techniques utilized, and the needed qualifications of the facilitators. This manuscript will discuss the findings of an intervention designed for African American couples and its impact on their relationship beliefs.

LITERATURE REVIEW

The field has recognized the need to develop healthy relationship interventions for African American couples (Larson, 2004; Sweeney & Phillips, 2004). The importance of understanding barriers experienced and the cultural context for African Americans and how to place these issues within a curriculum that can respond to these unique needs has been noted (Franklin, 2004; O'Connor, 2006). Healthy relationship education for African Americans must include a focus on (1) understanding sociocultural factors associated with marriage, (2) being knowledgeable of the historical factors that impact Black relationships, and (3) addressing resistance to marriage education (Franklin, 2004; Pinderhughes, 2002).

Relationships take place within a broader context that goes beyond the two partners and extends to families, communities and even the larger society (Bent-Goodley, 2011a; Hill, 1999). There are stereotypes of African American males and females that impact their ability to be in healthy relationships (Bent-Goodley, 2005a; Boyd-Franklin, 2006; Franklin, 2001). For example, African American women have been stereotyped as being sexually promiscuous, angry, overbearing, and unwilling to allow men to be men (Hill-Collins, 2008). They have also been stereotyped as being motherly in relationships and willing to accept whatever comes with being in the relationship. African American men have been stereotyped as unable to be in long-term relationships, lazy, hypermasculine, and violent (Hooks, 2003). These stereotypes have an impact on the relationship. The partners could have these negative stereotypes and could find themselves fighting against them or succumbing to them in the relationship. These negative stereotypes often come from media images, popular culture, and historical representations of African Americans.

There have also been discussions about the declining ratio of marriageable men in the Black community (Bent-Goodley, 2011a; O'Connor, 2006). The idea that Black women have fewer men to choose from for a relationship has created for some a sense of desperation and a willingness to tolerate things in a relationship that they would not ordinarily tolerate if there were more options of available men. On the other side, there is the idea that some men use this perception as an excuse for infidelity and to do things they know are wrong in the relationship. These issues are important to address in healthy relationship education.

The historical context has also been identified as being important. The idea that African Americans were not allowed to be in relationships during the enslavement of African people continues to be identified as significant to current relationship patterns today (Bent-Goodley, 2009; Franklin, 2001). The man-in-the-house rule was instituted so that any woman receiving public assistance in the 1960s would not be able to have a man living in the home (Bent-Goodley, 2011b; Franklin, 2001; Hill, 1999). This rule weakened and diminished the role of men as partners and fathers in the home. These issues continue to be identified as having an impact on Black male-female relationships today.

There is also a resistance to marriage education in the Black community, particularly among men (O'Conner, 2006). Marriage education is viewed as something that White people utilize and is not viewed as something that Black people utilize. In addition, talking about something so personal as an intimate relationship is further challenging to do when the person is forced to do so within other geographic and cultural communities and with people who do not look like them. There is also an impression that the professional community does not value the cultural context and understand how it impacts the relationship. Thus, there is a perception that marriage education will not work in the Black community.

OVERVIEW OF IN CIRCLE: A HEALTHY RELATIONSHIP INTERVENTION FOR AFRICAN AMERICAN COUPLES

In Circle was developed by and created for African American couples to learn about what constitutes a healthy relationship and to better understand how they can maintain a healthy relationship. The circle is symbolic in African culture. In essence, it means that the lives and the fate of people of African ancestry are all connected. Therefore, working together and resolving life's challenges not only benefits the individual but also serves to benefit the community. In Circle was created to promote healthy relationships, domestic violence prevention, and HIV risk behavior reduction. The intervention was developed with the support of a Community Advisory Board (CAB). The CAB reviewed different iterations of the intervention offering feedback and thinking about the intervention strengths and weaknesses. The content, structure, and delivery methods were reviewed and discussed with the CAB along with determining appropriate recruitment and retention methods to support the intervention. The CAB members reviewed the evaluation mechanisms to help assess the curriculum and also participated in the final event of the intervention to hear directly from the participants about their experience. Feedback was also obtained from two experts in the area of marriage education and cultural competence to ascertain their feedback and recommendations regarding the curriculum.

The In Circle curriculum is theory-based: guided by social cognitive theory, the ecological perspective, and the Afrocentric paradigm. Social cognitive theory views behavior from a non-pathological, non-victim-blaming stance (Lee, 2000). Essentially, this theory purports that if you can change the way one thinks about an issue or how one interprets an experience, then you can impact behavior (Bandura, 1999). Thus, intervention takes place largely within three domains: (1) engaging in cognitive restructuring, which includes identifying thinking patterns and revising false beliefs, (2) enhancing coping skills, which includes developing strategies to address problem situations and self-efficacy, and (3) developing problem-solving skills. Within a cultural context, social cognitive theory emphasizes that solutions need to be developed with a cultural lens that acknowledges the variation within groups and the need to focus on collective efficacy (Bandura, 1999, 2002). Related to this intervention, social cognitive theory was used to (1) frame the discussion on dispelling myths about domestic violence and HIV in the African American community in order to restructure thinking patterns about these issues, (2) to guide the sessions on enhancing coping strategies, and (3) to examine the use of problem-solving skills. The ecological perspective details the connections and intricacies of relationships and influences experienced by a single person within a larger environment (Abrams, Theberge, & Karan, 2005; Lee, 2000). This perspective acknowledges the larger environmental influences on behavior. Specific to this intervention, the ecological perspective was used to (1) identify internal and external stressors as they relate to environmental influences and barriers experienced by Black women and men, (2) identify positive stress management strategies, and (3) identify resources within the environment (Carlson, Furby, Armstrong, & Shlaes, 1997). The Afrocentric paradigm is a culturally specific framework that emphasizes core ethical principles within communities of African ancestry (Bent-Goodley, 2005b). Four essential principles of the Afrocentric paradigm include the need to focus on (1) the role of family structure, community connections, and the subjugation of individual needs to the larger familial and community needs, (2) the significance of spirituality as a means of coping and surviving life challenges, (3) the importance of the oral tradition to comprehend and translate information, and (4) the significance of using rituals to bind groups and contextualize experiences (Bent-Goodley, 2005b; Humphreys, 2000; Martin & Martin, 2002; Musgrave, Allen, & Allen, 2002). Specific to this intervention, (1) the group structure was used to foster a collective experience; (2) issues of secrecy and placing family and community first were discussed as they relate to the African American experience; (3) the community was involved through a CAB in program planning and implementation; (4) spirituality was affirmed and recognized as a part of each session; and, (5) building on the oral tradition, different mediums were used to support the intervention such as journaling, role-playing, and small-group discussions.

The Marriage Education Curriculum Assessment Guide (Hauer et al., 2008) was used as a framework to guide the process of creating the intervention. It was clear that the intervention had to include a focus on improving communication skills, resolving conflicts in a healthy manner, and focusing on commitment in the relationship (Adler-Baeder, Higginbotham, & Lamke, 2004; Jakubowski, Milne, Brunner, & Miller, 2004). There needed to be an in-depth exploration of a range of topics, and the impact and interaction with the social environment needed to be addressed (Hawkins, Carroll, Doherty, & Willoughby, 2004). The intervention needed to include a focus on addressing perceptions of marriage, how to sustain a healthy marriage, the idea that one must continue to work on maintaining a healthy relationship, the role of marriage in society, and the connection of marriage to the larger community (Halford et al., 2004). The curriculum also needed to use a variety of techniques for delivery, such as lectures, learning activities to be completed in the group and at home, role-playing, audio and video mechanisms, and interactive discussions (Hawkins et al., 2004). It was also important, from a cultural standpoint, to include storytelling as an opportunity to learn and hear diverse perspectives. This technique was added for that reason.

The intervention is rooted in the principles of Ma'at. The Principles of Ma'at are essentially seven value statements developed from ancient Egypt (Bent-Goodley, 2005a). These seven value statements or virtues form the basis for how one should think about themselves in relation to others in their community. It sets the tone for and provides the framework for the intervention. The seven principles are truth, justice, righteousness, order, balance, reciprocity, and harmony. Each of the principles was developed to guide important elements of the curriculum (Table 1).

The Principles of Ma'at, each of the seven virtues, were operationalized in each session to reflect a particular healthy relationship knowledge and skill set. Therefore, each session connects to one Principle of Ma'at for a total of seven sessions and seven principles covered. Session one was centered on the Virtue of Truth, which was operationalized as focusing on personal values, definitions, and expectations in a relationship. This session was centered on values clarification, understanding ones personal truths as it relates to expectations of a partner, relationship expectations generally and what constitutes a healthy relationship.

TABLE 1
Principles of Ma'at: The Seven Virtues

Principle or Virtue of Ma'at	Description
Truth	*I will always seek to know what is correct and I will not lie or speak falsely of myself, my family, my community or my race*
Justice	*I will always be fair in what I do and I will not cheat myself, my family, my community, or my race*
Righteousness	*I will always be correct in what I do and I will not allow others to influence me to do wrong to myself, my family or my race*
Order	*I will respect the natural order of the universe and I will not separate myself from that which gives order to myself, my family, my community, or my race*
Balance	*I will strive to understand and respect the need to be complimentary and I will not be in conflict with myself, my family, my community or my race*
Reciprocity	*I will always strive to do the proper thing at the right time and I will not bring shame to myself, my family, my community or my race*
Harmony	*I will always be in rhythm with what is good and I will never be in opposition to what is good for myself, my family, my community or my race*

Source: http://woodlawn.cps.k12.il.us/2_virtues.html

Session two was centered on the Virtue of Justice, which was operationalized as focusing on discussing definitions of domestic violence in the Black community, identifying signs of domestic violence, examining ways of managing conflict, and discerning between domestic violence and relationship conflict.

Session three was centered on the Virtue of Righteousness, which was operationalized as focusing on self-assessment and management. During this session, there was a focus on building self-management skills and discussing the role of empathy in a relationship. This session also provided information on building communication and problem-solving skills in a relationship.

Session four was centered on the Virtue of Order, which was operationalized as focusing on financial management. This session included a discussion of gender expectations related to money and finances and cultural considerations for African Americans and money management, including the importance of savings and investment planning. The session explored financial management and asset development and the meaning of money for Black couples, particularly when the woman makes more than the man or has a professional position compared to her partner's blue-collar position.

Session five was centered on the Virtue of Balance, which was operationalized as focusing on family roles and stress management. This session discussed the nature of gender roles and its impact on relationships. Types of parenting styles and the impact of fathering and mothering differently were discussed. In addition, the challenge of having multiple caregiving responsibilities was discussed particularly for individuals with responsibility for parents and children. The types and indicators of stress were discussed with healthy manners of managing such stress identified.

Session six was centered on the Virtue of Reciprocity, which was operationalized as focusing on intimacy and HIV prevention. During this session, couples discussed how to build trust in the relationship, and how intimacy looks different for men and women. Strategies of HIV prevention and safer sex were also discussed. In addition, the impact of the perception of having few marriageable men was discussed.

Session seven was centered on the Virtue of Harmony, which was operationalized as focusing on relationship management and maintenance. During this session, couples examined how issues of grief and loss impacted their relationships. Grief and loss were defined broadly to include father absence uniquely experienced by males and females. Methods of managing and maintaining relationships were also discussed. In addition, exploring ways of adapting to change in a relationship was examined.

The final session took place in the form of a closing ceremony, which focused on strengthening social support systems. In this final session, help-seeking strategies were discussed, and ways to strengthen social support networks were examined. Community members and board members were invited to attend the closing ceremony, which was done using African ceremonial rituals.

METHODS

Each couple participated in an eligibility screening to ensure that there was no domestic violence present in the relationship. Data were collected at two time points: a pretest self-administered prior to the start of the intervention and a posttest that was self-administered at the conclusion of the intervention. The primary outcomes of the curriculum were (1) to enhance knowledge of healthy relationships, (2) reduce exposure to domestic violence, and (3) increase knowledge of HIV risk and protective factors. This manuscript will report on the outcomes associated with improved knowledge of healthy relationships as evidenced through relationship beliefs.

The self-report instrument included measures on sociodemographic variables, relationship beliefs, exposure to domestic violence, mental health status, drug abuse, and sexual risk-taking behaviors. For the purposes of this manuscript, the demographic variables and data from the relationship beliefs measures will be discussed. The Relationship Belief Inventory (RBI) was used to understand beliefs and expectations about relationships. The reliability of the scale ranges from .58 to .83 (James, Hunsley, & Hemsworth, 2002). The RBI is a five eight-item scale examines communication patterns, conflict resolution, relationship expectations, and gender perceptions of needs. The RBI was used in previous marriage education research to include African American populations (Dunn & Schwebel, 1995).

RESULTS

The study consisted of 11 couples for a total of 22 people (Table 2). The majority were between the ages of 25 and 34 (64%), evenly distributed between ages 35 and 44 (14%) and 45 to 55 (14%), with the least amount between the ages of 18 and 24 (8%). The majority identified as African American (67%) and the remainder Caribbean American (33%). The majority were married (55%), over one-fourth were living together (27%), and nearly one-fifth were dating (18%). Over half of the sample had children (59%). The sample was well educated: master's degree (32%), high school diploma (27%), some graduate education (18%), some college (14%), and a college degree (9%). Most were employed (81%), students (14%), or unemployed (5%). In terms of income, 32% earned between $20,000 and $40,000, 31% earned under $20,000, 23% between $41,000 and $60,000, 9% between $61,000 and $80,000, and the remainder between $81,000 and $100,000 (5%). The majority of the couples were in their current relationship between 1 and 5 years (54%), 6 and 10 years (16%), 11 and 15 years (20%), and 16 and 20 years (10%). The majority of the participants belonged to a faith community (64%), and the remainder did not (36%). One-third had experienced at least one separation in their current relationship.

Table 3 presents the statistically significant findings in relationship beliefs at the pre- and posttest. There was a decline in participants who felt that *it is a personal insult when my partner disagrees with an important idea of mine.* Nearly one-third (32%) of the participants agreed with this statement at the pretest, and 18% agreed at the posttest ($p = .05$). At the pretest, 41% of the participants agreed with the statement that *men and women probably will never understand the opposite sex*; while, at posttest, 13% agreed with this statement ($p = .03$). There was an increase in agreement with the statement that *men and women need the same basic things out of a relationship* from the pretest (55%) to the posttest (68%) ($p = .03$). At the pretest, 55% of the participants agreed with the statement that *I cannot tolerate it when my partner argues with me*; while 44% agreed with this statement at the posttest ($p = .05$). There was an increase in agreement with the statement that *if my sexual partner does not get satisfied completely, it does not mean that I have failed* from the pretest (59%) to the posttest (82%; $p = .03$). There was a decrease in agreement with the statement that *when my partner and I disagree, I feel like our relationship is falling apart* from pretest (28%) to posttest (13%; $p = .05$). There was an increase in agreement with the statement that *if you don't like the way a relationship is going, you can make it better* from pretest (82%) to posttest (100%; $p = .03$).

Limitations

There are a number of limitations with regard to this study. First, the sampling strategy used a convenience sample approach, and the participants self-selected to participate. Therefore, the findings cannot be generalized to broader populations. Also, the sample size was small, which did not allow for multivariate-level analysis. Despite these limitations, the findings point to an intervention that has promise with responding to the unique challenges faced by African American couples in relationships.

TABLE 2
Selected Demographic Characteristics of Study Participants

Selected Demographic Characteristics	N	%
Age		
18–24	2	8%
25–34	14	64%
35–44	3	14%
45–54	3	14%
Gender		
Male	11	50%
Female	11	50%
Race/ethnicity		
African American	15	67%
Caribbean American	7	33%
Marital status		
Married	12	55%
Living together	6	27%
Dating	4	18%
Children		
Yes	13	59%
No	9	41%
Education		
High school	6	27%
Some college	3	14%
College degree	2	9%
Some graduate education	4	18%
Master's degree	7	32%
Income		
Under $20,000/yr	7	31%
$21,000–$40,000/yr	7	32%
$41,000–$60,000/yr	5	23%
$61,000–$80,000/yr	2	9%
$81,000–$100,000/yr	1	5%
Length of time in relationship		
1–5 years	12	54%
6–10 years	4	16%
11–15 years	6	20%
16–20 years	2	10%
Employment status		
Employed	18	81%
Unemployed	1	5%
Student	3	14%
Separation in past year		
Yes	7	33%
No	15	67%
Belonged to a church		
Yes	14	64%
No	8	36%

TABLE 3
Relationship Beliefs

Variable	Pretest (n = 22)	Posttest (n = 22)	X^2, p value
Personal insult	32%	18%	17.00, $p = .05$
Opposite sex	41%	13%	16.00, $p = .03$
Same basic things	55%	68%	16.00, $p = .03$
Tolerate	55%	44%	16.94, $p = .05$
Sexual partner	59%	82%	14.06, $p = .03$
Disagree	28%	13%	17.00, $p = .05$
Make it better	82%	100%	16.00, $p = .03$
Tuned in	19%	6%	16.00, $p = .03$
Mysteries	59%	37%	17.00, $p = .05$

Discussion

The focus of this manuscript was to share findings of how the In Circle intervention impacted relationship beliefs among African American couples. The intervention did show an improvement in more positive relationship beliefs at the conclusion of the intervention. The participants evidenced a better understanding of the value of communication in relationships and the importance of sharing expectations in a relationship. They also were less likely at the end of the intervention to think that the other gender was a mystery or could not be figured out. In addition, they were able to make more connections between similar needs across gender in relationships, particularly in the areas of communication and managing conflict. They were able to understand that a relationship requires work and that one cannot be in a relationship without being prepared to consistently invest time and energy in maintaining the relationship. The participants also evidenced more awareness about what takes place in a healthy relationship. They had a more positive outlook about the nature of disagreements in relationships and learned not to personalize disagreements but instead to view them as opportunities for further discussion and communication. Finally, the findings point to a greater awareness of the value of having a positive self-perception to avoid negatively or inappropriately personalizing issues that arise in the relationship.

Implications

It is important to design healthy relationship education initiatives that speak to the cultural context of individuals receiving the intervention. By developing interventions that are conceptually and intentionally designed for a group, one can create opportunities for improved beliefs about relationships and what constitutes a healthy relationship. The In Circle intervention is undergoing further testing with a larger sample to determine its efficacy and effectiveness as an intervention. The value of creating such interventions within the Black community is very important.

Working with the faith-based community to implement healthy relationship education can be positive. When conducting such an intervention in partnership with the faith-based community, one is able to draw upon a diverse group of African Americans ethnically, socially, and economically. The church provided a safe place to have the conversation about relationships in an environment that had integrity and trust from the population, even among those who did not belong to a faith-based community. In addition, it included individuals who often do not turn to social service providers for support. Thus, placing the intervention within the community and in partnership with a trusted entity encouraged diversity among the study population compared to what is seen in traditional research.

The African American Healthy Marriage Initiative provides an important vehicle to advance discussions regarding policy needs for African American couples and families. Maintaining such an initiative within the federal government is important to bring attention to the broader, social, political, and economic issues impacting African American couples. Policies to support income and wealth development in the African American community are important to supporting African American couples. Financial issues continue to profoundly impact African American couples. Addressing disparities in income, employment, and wealth is important to sustaining African American marriages and relationships. Policies that provide resources for increased domestic violence and HIV prevention awareness and intervention in the African American community are also needed.

The In Circle intervention needs to be tested within a larger sample of African American couples to move it toward an evidence-based model for healthy marriage intervention. In addition, funding strategies should be maintained and augmented to conduct research related to marriage and healthy relationship education for African American couples. Current funding is inconsistent and often limited. These additional supports are needed to use the research to solidify and expand interventions for African American families and couples.

CONCLUSION

African American couples have an interest in learning more about how to preserve and sustain their relationships. When given a geographically accessible and culturally sensitive intervention option, they readily participated and were able to expand upon their relationship beliefs around what is needed to support a healthy relationship. In Circle evidences promise in helping to inform African American couples of relationships and to impact their thinking about themselves within the relationship.

REFERENCES

Abrams, K., Theberge, S. K., & Karan, O. C. (2005). Children and adolescents who are depressed: An ecological approach. *Professional School Counseling, 8*(3), 284–293.

Adler-Baeder, F., Higginbotham, B., & Lamke, L. (2004). Putting empirical knowledge to work: Leading research and programming on marital quality. *Family Relations, 53*, 537–546.

Bandura, A. (1999). A social cognitive theory of personality. In L. Pervin & O. P. John (Eds.), *Handbook of personality: Theory and research* (2nd ed., pp. 154–196). New York, NY: Guilford Publications.

Bandura, A. (2002). Social cognitive theory in cultural context. *Applied Psychology: An International Review, 151*, 269–290.

Bent-Goodley, T. B. (2005a). Culture and domestic violence: Transforming knowledge development. *Journal of Interpersonal Violence, 20*, 195–203.

Bent-Goodley, T. B. (2005b). An African centered approach to domestic violence. *Families in Society, 86*, 197–206.

Bent-Goodley, T. B. (2009). A Black experience-based approach to gender-based violence. *Social Work, 54*, 262–269.

Bent-Goodley, T. B. (2011a). *The ultimate betrayal: A renewed perspective of domestic violence.* Washington, DC: NASW Press.

Bent-Goodley, T. B. (2011b). Regulating the lives of children: Kinship care as a cultural resistance of the African American community. In J. Schiele (Ed.), *Social welfare policy: Regulation and resistance among people of color* (pp. 25–42). Thousand Oaks, CA: Sage Publications.

Bent-Goodley, T. B. (Ed.). (in press). *By grace: The challenges, promise and strengths of Black marriages.* Washington, DC: NASW Press.

Bent-Goodley, T. B., & Williams, O. J. (2008). *Community insights on domestic violence among African Americans: Conversations about domestic violence and other issues affecting their community, Detroit, Michigan.* St. Paul, MN: Institute on Domestic Violence in the African American Community.

Blackman, L., Clayton, O., Glenn, N., Malone-Colon, L., & Roberts, A. (2005). *The consequences of marriage for African Americans: A comprehensive literature review*. New York, NY: Institute for American Values.

Boyd-Franklin, N. (2006). *Black family therapy: Understanding the African American experience* (2nd ed.). New York, NY: Guilford.

Brotherson, S., & Duncan, W. (2004). Rebinding the ties that bind: Government efforts to preserve and promote marriage. *Family Relations, 53*, 459–468.

Carlson, E. B., Furby, L., Armstrong, J., & Shlaes, J. (1997). A conceptual framework for the long-term psychological effects of traumatic childhood abuse. *Child Maltreatment: Journal of the American Professional Society on the Abuse of Children, 93*, 272–295.

Dakin, K. J., & Wampfer, R. (2008). Money doesn't buy happiness, but it helps: Marital satisfaction, psychological distress, and demographic differences between low and middle income clinic couples. *The American Journal of Family Therapy, 36*, 300–311.

Doherty, W., & Anderson, J. (2004). Community marriage initiatives. *Family Relations, 53*, 425–432.

Dunn, R. L., & Schwebel, A. I. (1995). Meta-analytic review of mantal therapy outcome research. *Journal of Family Psychology, 9*, 58–68.

Franklin, D. L. (2001). *What's love got to do with it? Understanding and healing the rift between black men and women*. New York, NY: Simon & Schuster.

Franklin, R. M. (2004). *Healthy marriages in low-income African-American communities: A thematic summary*. Baltimore, MD: Annie E. Casey Foundation.

Halford, W., Moore, E., Wilson, K., Farrugia, C., & Dyer, C. (2004). Benefits of flexible delivery relationship education: An evaluation of the Couple CARE Program. *Family Relations, 53*, 469–476.

Hauer, J., McDowell, L., Andrews, B., Swanson, L., Marr, P., & Minor, B. (2008). *Marriage education curriculum assessment guide*. Washington, DC: U.S. Department of Health and Human Services Administration for Children and Families.

Hawkins, A. Carroll, J., Doherty, W., & Willoughby, B. (2004). A comprehensive framework for marriage education. *Family Relations, 53*, 547–558.

Hill, R. (1999). *The strengths of African American families: Twenty-five years later.* Lanham, MD: The University Press of America.

Hill-Collins, P. (2008). *Black feminist thought: Knowledge, consciousness, and the politics of empowerment*. New York, NY: Routledge.

Hooks, B. (2003). *We real cool: Black men and masculinity*. New York, NY: Routledge.

Humphreys, J. (2000). Spirituality and distress in sheltered battered women. *Journal of Nursing Scholarship, 32*, 273–278.

Jakubowski, S. F., Milne, E. P., Brunner, H., & Miller, R. B. (2004). A review of empirically supported marital enrichment programs. *Family Relations, 53*, 528–536.

James, S., Hunsley, J., & Hemsworth, D. (2002). Factor structure of the Relationship Belief Inventory. *Cognitive Therapy and Resaerch, 26*, 729–744.

Larson, J. (2004). Innovations on marriage education: Introduction and challenges. *Family Relations, 53*, 421–424.

Lee, M. Y. (2000). Understanding Chinese battered women in North America: A review of the literature and practice implications. *Journal of Multicultural Social Work, 8*, 215–241.

Martin, E. P., & Martin, J. M. (2002). Spirituality and the Black helping tradition in social work. Washington, DC: NASW Press.

Musgrave, C., Allen, C., & Allen, G. (2002). Spirituality and health for women of color. *American Journal of Public Health, 92*, 557–560.

O'Connor, V. (2006, February). *Barriers to marriage and parenthood for African American men and women*. Syracuse, NY: Syracuse University.

Pinderhughes, E. (2002). African American marriage in the 20th century. *Family Process, 41*, 269–282.

Sweeney, M., & Phillips, J. (2004). Understanding racial differences in marital disruption: Recent trends and explanations. *Journal of Marriage and Family, 66*, 639–650.

Arab American Marriage: Culture, Tradition, Religion, and the Social Worker

Alean Al-Krenawi

Achva Academic College and Spitzer Department of Social Work, Ben-Gurion University of the Negev, Beer-Sheva, Israel

Stephen O. Jackson

Department of Education, Memorial University of Newfoundland, St. John's, Newfoundland, Canada

The growing and varied Arab American population and the continuing stereotyping and mistrust between people of Arab descent and other Americans make the need for culturally competent social work more pronounced. This study considers the importance the institutions of marriage and family retain within what can be a generally high-context community. Marriage, family, and religious relationships can be complicated by a sense of honor and stigma alongside frequently distressing experiences or news from the country of origin. Various generations of Arab Americans are returning with their Middle Eastern counterparts to their religions to reestablish their identities. We shall consider the problems between fundamental and enlightened readings and understandings of the traditional marriage contract, especially under Sharia law, and traditional gender roles in relation to the varied expectations of the bride and groom, the extended families, and the cultural community. We suggest ways that social workers can develop skillful communications within effective cultural community networks to offset both inappropriate and insensitive misdiagnosis and treatment.

INTRODUCTION

More than 10 years after 9/11 and almost 2 years after the Arab Spring, many Americans still have profound fears, stereotypes, and misunderstandings of Arab Americans. So too do many Arab people sometimes fear or mistrust the intentions of many American peoples. Western-trained social workers must address these misunderstandings, open the doors to communication, and attempt to know and understand people of differing backgrounds; the problems each face in understanding themselves and their world. The growing and ever-changing political, national, and cultural aspirations of Middle Eastern peoples have a profound impact upon people of Arab descent in America—whether they are new immigrants or visitors or whether their family has been in America for generations. Social workers and other helping professionals are challenged by the rejuvenated hopes and dreams of men, women, and children who are dealing with conflicting identities, purposes, and allegiances. Practitioners must prepare to accept and reconcile cultural differences and nuances, as they would with any other person, so they might provide effective services to people of Arab origin.

Though hard statistics are difficult to determine, there are likely over 5 million people of Arab descent in America based upon both the 2000 census and more current figures of Muslim and Christian communities in America (Abu Baker, 2003; Arab American Association, n.d.; Gearing et al., 2013; Hodge, 2005; Soheilian & Inman, 2009). The majority have been born in the United States and, despite common attempts to label or stereotype, are not racially distinct from White North Americans, nor do they represent any singular traditional *type*. They may share the same language and a similar culture, but there are different ethnic streams. An Arab is not simply a Muslim; there are many Arab people of different religions. The Muslim populations of Turkey, Afghanistan, Pakistan, and Sudan are not considered Middle Eastern or Arab. Most Muslims in the United States are South Asian or African American. Arab people have come from all over the Middle East and live mainly in urban centers, with 66% distributed through 10 states alone: 33% live in California, Michigan, and New York/New Jersey (Arab American Association, n.d.; Erickson & Al-Timimi, 2001; Padela & Heiser, 2010).

Most Arab Americans are Christian (Arfken, Kubiak, & Koch, 2007, p. 610), though this ratio is changing considerably (Erickson & Al-Timimi, 2001; Hodge, 2005). Arab Muslims follow two main types of Islam: *Sunni* (main) and *Shia*. Arab Christian people can be Maronite Catholic, Melkite Catholic, Syrian Catholic, Chaldean Catholic, Roman Catholic, Antiochian Orthodox, Syrian Orthodox, Coptic Orthodox, or Protestant (Abudabbeh, 2005; Arab American Association, n.d.). Some Arab people find that with such similarities in lifestyle and attitudes, religious beliefs and the specific interpretations or nuances of each can often be their main distinguishing or identifying feature (Erickson & Al-Timimi (2001). Abudabbeh (2005) suggests that Christian Arabs "often impress outsiders as being more 'Arab' than Muslims. It is not uncommon to find Arab Christians holding traditional and conventional attitudes towards a variety of issues synonymous to those held by Muslim Arab Americans" (p. 425). We have mentioned similarities in religious orthodoxies and, conversely, there are many secular Muslims who still believe in the tenets of Islam but not necessarily in its primacy over all other rules of law (Armstrong, 1993). So while our main religious discussion will regard Islam, the traditional elements related to marriage, gender relationships, and the family will resound through many other people of Arab heritage.

Up to 85% of Arab Americans hold a high school diploma, while almost 40% hold a degree from a university. Nearly twice as many Arab Americans have a graduate degree than the national average. Arab American families tend to make more money than the national average, with 30% having an annual income of over $75,000 compared to the national average of 22% (Abudabbeh, 2005; Arab American Association, n.d.). While immigration laws give preference to people with higher education and economic standing, this also reflects the strong ambition within Arab cultures to maintain honor through good education and financial independence (Arab American Association, n.d.; Erickson & Al-Timimi, 2001; Hodge, 2005). As of 2005, 57% of Arab Americans were married as opposed to the national average (54%), while less were currently divorced (Kayyali, 2006, p. 75).

With the growth of the Arab population in America, particularly those coming from Muslim backgrounds, there is a need for cultural competency in social work. This is not a new idea of course, but Boyle & Springer (2001) suggest that this often still seems to be an ideal rather than a measureable practice. For example, while the first attempts to provide culturally competent assistance to children with emotional problems took place in the 1980s (Hurdle, 2002), it was not until 2008 that the National Association of Social Workers officially revised their directive in their code of ethics to suggest that

Social workers should obtain education about and seek to understand the nature of social diversity and oppression with respect to race, ethnicity, national origin, color, sex, sexual orientation, gender identity or expression, age, marital status, political belief, religion, immigration status, and mental or physical disability. (Urban and Lund, 2010; National Association of Social Workers, 2008)

In 2002, The White House instituted a Commission on Complementary and Alternative Medicine that recommended the integration of alternative health care practices into regular professional practice, a profoundly important aspect of caring for many Arab Americans; in many Arab countries, religious imams are employed by hospitals to complement medical services (Abu-Ras, 2007; Boyle and Springer, 2001). The key word here was *complementary* as the board took pains to state that, while there is an indicated need and desire to practice alternative forms of social work and psychiatric therapies, there are often few concrete plans for working with people originally of other cultures, nor is there the empirical scientific knowledge to legitimate the use of certain practices to administrative heads who often lack the know-how to institute some of these ideas (Ben-Arye et al., 2009; Boyle and Springer, 2001; Erickson & Al-Timimi, 2001).

This lack might explain why, in a recent review of literature on the subject of social work and mental health intervention with Arab families, which would include considerable dealing with marital and familial conflicts, Gearing et al. (2013) found 78 potential barriers and challenges to productive social work: 42.5% of them because of misunderstanding the cultural context. Hodge (2005) found that 86% of Muslim respondents in the United States felt it important that counselors should have an understanding of Islamic principles.

Here we intend to familiarize the practitioner with some basic elements of Arab cultures that might be found within a recent immigrant or someone who has been in America for some time. We shall include some of the basic tenets of marriage, the male/female gender roles and relationships, and the importance of maintaining strong families in the Arab tradition. There is both a strong religious and a strong traditional background to this, important to note because we find the renewal of marriage and family structure with religious sanction are becoming more important elements to asserting especially Arab Muslim identities. We shall consider some of the problems that seem to be inherent in the marital and gender relationships that have led to conflicts between asserting *Arabic, regular, or fundamentalist, Christian or Islamic* identities versus more *Westernized* identities. There is a schizophrenia that may develop within Arab Americans who are looking for acceptance, and we should discuss whether and how these are being addressed within and without Islam. Finally, we shall consider some ideas that might contribute to best practices for social workers, particularly when dealing with marital and familial problems.

ARAB CULTURE

High Context

Many Arab people can be defined as being high context in that the person is highly influenced by the family, community, and institutions that surround them:

High-context cultures tend to emphasize the collective over the individual, have a slower pace of social change, and tend to value social stability. Low-context cultures tend to emphasize the individual over the collective, have a faster pace of social change, and tend to value social flux rather than stability.... (Al-Krenawi & Graham, 2005, p. 302)

An understanding of the collectivist identity can illuminate the integral relationship between a person and the group, the nature of authority and family authority, the pressure of community demands upon its members, and the importance of doing ones part and saving face within the community (Abu Baker, 2003). The use of the term *community* in this paper will most often refer to the cultural community.

Where low-context cultures tend to be more egalitarian in structure, high-context cultures tend to be more hierarchical, highly patriarchal, and pyramidal (Al-Krenawi & Graham, 2005; Dwairy et al., 2006). "Although families may have established their own households, they nevertheless maintain the concept of extension by considering their own kin of being worthy of the most attention, of being confided in, and of their allegiance" (Abudabbeh, 2005, p. 427). Marriage is an alliance of families, and members of each family will provide loyalty, emotional support, and even financial assistance to each other rather than simply to the bride and groom (Al-Krenawi, 2005a; Erickson & Al-Timimi, 2001). The marriage is usually arranged and, while the arrangement is supposed to be acceptable to the bride and groom, their opinion can often be overlooked (Abudabbeh, 2005). The practice of marriage between first cousins is still practiced, though much less often, because cousins rather than *outsiders* can often provide a more reliable, and cheaper, alliance (Abudabbeh, 2005; Al-Krenawi, Graham, Dean, & Eltaiba, 2004).

The community or family will also decide where you live, what career you will pursue, and other important decisions. Most people do not leave home until they are married. Even then, they may live close by, if not in extensions to family abodes. Many Arab people are discouraged from committing crimes or other misbehaviors such as substance abuse, sexual deviance, or other dalliances not just for religious reasons but for fear of stigmatization in the family and community. Family problems are expected to be dealt with in private—quickly and quietly (Abudabbeh, 2005; Al-Krenawi & Graham, 2005; Arfken, Kubiak, & Farrag, 2009; Bradley, 2010; Erikson and Al-Timimi, 2001; Soheilian & Inman, 2009). Otherwise, religious and other community institutions will provide the first source of identification and treatment of problems (Al-Krenawi & Graham, 2003).

Dwairy (2006) suggests that the collective tradition dates back to when Arab tribes needed the security within their own ranks to ensure survival against others. To remain strong, authority would have to be rigid, with each part of the community doing its share of both the work and organization. The family is the unit of strength that could perpetuate the strength of the whole (Al-Krenawi & Graham, 2005). Such strong allegiances and dependencies have remained in many parts of the Middle East despite the variances of interpretation and socioeconomic changes that have taken place. The introduction of various religions into this structure have changed understandings of individuality, for example, but the Islamic principles especially served only to extend the ideas of collectivity beyond simple tribal lines to more universal communities; we see the growth of the universal Islamic Ummah alongside smaller Christian Brotherhoods and the like. With the revival of Islam and of many other nationalist sentiments from the Arab Spring, we see also the revival of the importance of family and community as *keepers of the faith*, unlike what we might see in lower context American families (Abudabbeh, 2005; Armstrong. 1993). The family remains a source of strength for many Arab Americans who may feel marginalized in *everyday* American society.

Gender Roles and Duties: Religion and Tradition

There are strong expectations of both the mother and father within a family, and the loss of either one can affect the family profoundly. It is important to know of the generally accepted duties of most wives and the importance that both men and women place upon them. A wife is supposed to have and nurture babies. It is hoped that one will be a boy to continue the family name. Many women still do not work outside the home (Al-Krenawi, 2013). A mother is often responsible for the first nurturing of religious observance and orthodoxy among the children. At least in name and definition, the mother's role is considered the most revered in the family and the community (Abu-Ras, 2007; Al-Krenawi et al., 2004).

Despite *Western* feeling that many Arab women are oppressed, Erickson & Al-Timimi (2001) imply that a wife and mother can exert influence in ways that we may not see—by withholding her work and her favor perhaps until the husband and children show her more respect. Mahmood (2005), for example, suggests that some Arab women promote a more fundamental Islamic stance and demand that her husband also be more devout rather than pursue the less responsible and more un-Islamic, philandering stance that some Arab men adopt (Al-Krenawi & Graham, 2005).

Generally, men in Arab society are expected to be strong and not show signs of weakness. In times of family stress, they will assist in helping others but rarely seek help for themselves (Al-Krenawi & Graham, 2005). "Women's lives are an ongoing process of negotiating [this] ... patriarchal context" (Al-Krenawi & Graham, 2005, p. 302). Women are encouraged to remain docile and complacent at all times, even while they are told to give up their paychecks and similar vestiges of independence (Abu Baker, 2006; Al-Krenawi & Graham, 2005). Rather than forcing a man to admit to sterility, a woman will do so in his place, even as this may consequently be used as a social excuse to get a new *fertile* wife (Al-Krenawi & Graham, 2005). Men will limit women's mobility to protect their virtue: Courtships are strictly monitored, and an unmarried woman must still be looked after by male family members rather than gain independence in another abode (Erickson & Al-Timimi, 2001).

Interpreting Religion

Abudabbeh (2005) suggests that the family is the body of the Arab person while Islam and the Qur'an, for Muslims, are the soul (p. 426). However, religion in general can often be blamed for motivating marriage traditions or practices that are in fact part of cultural heritage rather than religion. It is important for a practitioner to be clear on the main principles of Islam and Christianity, as both can be misinterpreted and, rightly or wrongly, blamed for motivating violent and destructive activity (Al-Krenawi & Graham, 2005). Both the Qur'an and the Bible provide specific directions for the way people should live their lives, from birth to marriage to death. In some cases, they also include punishment for certain sins that can be committed between husband, wife, and family and within other social quarters. We shall see shortly that, while many suggested these dictates were originally meant as at least rudimentary forms of justice, peace, and equality within what was a more lawless world, unfortunate misinterpretations or the ideas of *taqlid* (returning to original practice) can sometimes lead to the terrible treatment of women, children, detractors, and others (Armstrong, 1993; Denny, 2006).

In general, the myriad understandings of Christianity and Islam fall into more literal or *textualist* understandings versus more liberal or critical interpretations (Al Krenawi, 2005a). In Sharia law, the words in the Qur'an are considered primary. When this comes to marriage, it is important then to understand the words in the Qur'an said to have been revealed to the prophet Muhammad. This would be considered the Qur'anic tradition, the basic ideals that most people of Islam would wish to live up to. When we speak of the difficulties encountered from this, we shall speak of the interpretations of these words that have all intended toward achieving an ideal state yet led to different understandings and applications (Yamani, 2008).

The interpretations of Islam are further guided by Hadiths: stories of how Mohammed lived his life as an exemplary Muslim (the Christian counterpart might be parables, though there are differences). These seek to clarify through a story questions not answered specifically in the Qur'an. There was fractionalization very early in the history of Islam, with a major rift happening just after Muhammad's death and a series of *fitnas* (chaotic periods), which resulted in many schools of thought for each of, for example, the Sunni, Shia, and Druze sects of Islam (Armstrong, 1993; Denny, 2006). Thus, as with parables, there are arguments over the validity of some hadiths, just as there are great arguments over translations of the original languages by scholars who are trying to be the most accurate they can be, to modernize interpretations, or to prove different ideas (Armstrong, 1993; Denny, 2006). However, in Arab countries, Sharia law becomes even more complicated as problems that are not covered in either the Qur'an or the hadiths are now subject to further decisions from religious councils who consult, make, and record *fiqh* (legal decisions). With new decisions, we hear of official religious pronouncements such as *fatwas*: a word that simply means a decision or ruling, but which has carried ominous overtones for Westerners who hear of the threatening *fatwas* from violent fundamentalists.

Importantly, Sharia Law in Islam, as with Christianity in some cases, is considered by many to trump the civil law of the land. Some may claim their destructive activity to be sacrosanct dependent on how they interpret their religion (Abu-Odeh, 2004). The practitioner may find people who follow the dictates of marriage and family responsibility in accordance with Sharia law and in defiance of accepted civil laws. However, rather than simply condemn this practice, the practitioner should also understand how complicated clients feel it can be to juxtapose civil and religious understandings. Muslims rites of marriage can be quite specific and, when followed too literally, can lead to many practices not normally condoned in American jurisprudence.

Religion, Rights, and Freedom in Marriage

It should be made clear that there are differing views of freedom between people, whether Arab or otherwise. Within many high-context communities, there is the idea that freedom is the ability to act the best way you can within the confines of your gender and social situation. Therefore, a person has rights, but they are in context to the community as a whole; they are not individualized. A sense of liberation comes from being given strict religious and societal guidelines and thus knowing where personal freedoms can be negotiated (Abu-Odeh, 2004; Elsaidi, 2011; Geertz, 2009; Kuran, 2009; Sidani & Thornberry, 2009).

More importantly today, marriage is considered by many to be an example of the strength of Arab, mainly Islamic, culture against a more decadent *Western* society (Fargues, 2001). Many people working for women's rights in the Arab world still see it possible to accomplish more rights and freedoms within the confines of enlightened religious thinking known as *itjihad* (Abu-Odeh, 2004; Al-Hibri, 1997). Abu-Odeh summarizes the debate well:

> Islam, the West, and patriarchy represent the defining ends of the triangle within ... feminism.... Toward each it has developed a response. In relation to the first (Islam), it is modernizing (when its interlocutor is a religious adversary). In relation to the second (the West), it is an apologist (when its interlocutor is Western). In relation to the third (patriarchy), it is liberal. (p. 199)

Fundamentalism as specifically a reaction to *Western* ideals will be considered again. Castells (2010) says specifically that

> Islamic fundamentalism is not a traditionalist movement. For all the efforts of exegesis to root Islamic identity in history and the holy texts, Islamists proceeded, for the sake of social resistance and political insurgency, with a reconstruction of cultural identity that is in fact hypermodern. (p. 17)

Here it is difficult to separate patriarchy from religion. Men in particular are losing control of identity in an atmosphere that seems hostile or seems to demand conformity to certain ideals. Appadurai (2006) discusses how these types of borderless nationalisms can develop to identify people in ways that oppose a state they feel is repressing them. We must closely consider all variables as to how Arab Americans view the blend of their own rights, religion, fundamentalism, and marriage.

Love versus Family versus Freedom

Yamani (2008) sums up the purpose of marriage for Muslims: "The main purpose of marriage in Islam is long-term cohabitation, procreation, the satisfaction of physical needs and the need for companionship that God has created within humanity" (p. 77). As with many religions, then, Islam dictates that sexual relationships between men and women are reserved for marriage. This idea can be a justification for controlling relationships, and especially dating or courting, between men and women. There is the traditional fear that a woman may tempt or fall prey to a man's physiological lack of control and aggressive advances. Sabry (2010), however, decries this as an anti-human sentiment that more Muslim people seem to be acknowledging: People seem to vilify those who cross personal and sexual boundaries, suggesting that true and free individual love between a man and a woman is as unmanageable and unwanted as a sexual encounter between them.

Of course, love exists within and without marriages, and though there is not much talk of love between men and women in religion, more Muslim brides and grooms are insisting that it must exist for marriage to be considered (Hoodfar, 2009). More women and men do not wish to marry before their education is complete, and in fact some young women and men may try to recruit more understanding, *loving* spouses through social circles in colleges and so forth rather than allow the family to choose a spouse (Fargues, 2001; Hoodfar, 2009). Many others do not feel arranged marriages should be circumvented: There are many stories where women whose husbands tend to stray later from their financial and family duties suggest that they might have been better off marrying more wisely than out of love alone (Fargues, 2001; Hoodfar, 2009).

Many Arab people negatively judge unmarried women and, to avoid such stigma being projected onto the family as a whole, parents may push young females into marriage at an early age also to solidify an alliance and avoid the woman becoming *undesirable* (Abu Baker, 2003). This is not entirely unwelcome as many young women, recognizing that their status and independence will increase at marriage, will accept marriage as a means to leave the family's strict confines. Women may prefer to marry older men who might display more intellectual and emotional maturity as opposed to having to adopt a mother role to a young, still coddled husband (Sidani & Thornberry, 2009).

The marriage contract often lays out exactly what obligations the bride and groom will have to each other: whether the woman will be allowed to work, whether she must wear *hijab*, how much the man is to contribute to the family financially, and other such guidelines. At times, the guardian (*wali*) may try to commandeer more dowry or discourage the marriage because the woman has lucrative work (Yamani, 2008). Whatever the conditions, these contracts may become very complex, often defining rigid gender roles that civil law would not necessarily enforce. Indeed, one of the spouses may be brought from the home country precisely because of these different traditions or understandings (Ferguson, 2004). However it turns out, the families, both in America and in the home country, and perhaps the cultural communities will take such agreements seriously (Hoodfar, 2009; Yamani, 2008). That having been said, these contract rules are also being used more recently to negotiate conditions that may liberate women from certain traditional expectations that might normally be enforced (Hoodfar, 2009; Yamani, 2008).

We can note that not all parts of a contract will be honored by certain Sharia courts if they go against a particular interpretation of Islam. Unfortunately, these are usually the ones that give more freedom to women and question the dominion of men over their families (Hoodfar, 2009; Yamani, 2008). We begin to see where clashes occur between traditional, fundamentalist, and liberal or enlightened thinking occur. We shall now consider some main parts of Arab Islamic marriage to provide examples.

Dowry, Duties, Woman as Property, Remaining Chaste, Punishment

A special note should be made here: When considering quotations from the Qur'an, we should remember again that there are slightly different translations or interpretations through the different schools. Those quoted lines in parentheses are often the additions of certain scholars and may be said a little differently by someone else. The purpose is to demonstrate the potential for problematic interpretations and to lay the foundation for current thinking on the subject.

Two passages from the Qur'an support the payment of a dowry: Surah 4.4, says to "give to the women (*whom you marry*) their (*Mahr dowry*) ... with a good heart ... " (Al-Hilali & Khan, 1996). The second Surah 4.24 says to the man that

> [a]ll women ... are lawful to you provided you seek them with your wealth in modest conduct, not in fornication.... All others are lawful, provided you seek them in marriage with *Mahr* ... for your property, desiring chastity, not committing illegal sexual intercourse, so with those of whom you have enjoyed sexual relations, give them their *Mahr* as prescribed ... (Al-Hilali & Khan, 1996)

Three things arise: First, a man must marry a woman to have sexual relations; second, if you have already had sexual relations, you must marry them; third, and more controversial today, is that the woman is to be had as chaste property. Muslim men and women may tend to take these verses seriously more regularly than people of other religions. Of course, there are similar verses and understandings in other religions, the spirit that can be seen in other people's marriages; these lines do not necessarily reflect the spirit of American jurisprudence (Armstrong, 1993).

This latter idea of the woman as sexual property is mentioned earlier, in Surah 2.223, which suggests that "Your wives are *tilth* for you, so go to your *tilth*, when or how you will, and send (good deeds, or ask Allah to bestow upon you pious offspring) for your own selves beforehand" (Al-Hilali & Khan, 1996). The word *tilth* is defined in this copy of the Qur'an as "sexual relations in a specific manner as to procreate and not deviant from that." Marriage contracts will assume at least that each party is agreeing to serve the physical needs of the other party; however, this is with the idea that a woman may only have one man (and there is no mention of physical enjoyment) while the husband may have up to four women (which we will discuss shortly). In exchange, the man is expected to take care of his wife (Yamani, 2008).

We can notice the beginnings of problems, as obedience begins to be measured in everything including sexual performance and giving birth, and the responsibility of a man begins to be dependent on whether his wife obeys. Worse is the tendency for some people to accept the dictates of Surah 4.32 (similar lines exist in other religious texts) that suggest that "men are the protector and maintainers of women" because they are better than the other and spend their income to support them. Righteous women must be devoutly obedient and guard their chastity and their husband's property. Those women who misbehave should first be admonished, then be sent to bed alone. If all that fails, they should be beaten (Surah 4.32; Al-Hilali & Khan, 1996; Yamani, 2008).

A further verse that severely dictates who should be married and warns against any liaison before or after marriage is found in Surah 4.25:

> ... so marry them with the permission of their masters, and give them their dowries justly, they being chaste, not fornicating, nor receiving paramours; and when they are taken in marriage, then if they are guilty of indecency, they shall suffer half the punishment which is (inflicted) upon free women. (Al-Hilali & Khan, 1996)

Again, Armstrong (1993) suggests that while these lines may have initially tried to temper more outrageous treatment of women in particular, literalist interpretations of the Qur'an reflect strictly patriarchal traditions that have killed that original spirit. Castells (2010) agrees that these fundamentalist readings of both Islamic and Christian verses are the result of an overall breakdown in traditional patriarchal society and resulting crises in male identity.

That a person, particularly a woman, practices chastity, takes care in receiving *paramours*, and dresses appropriately are hardly peculiar to any one particular religious group; it is a debate that possibly all Americans of all backgrounds have had. However, some people find it difficult to detach violent aspects in one part of these lines from others (Castells, 2010; Abu-Odeh, 2004; Al-Hibri, 1997). Terrible verbal, physical, and sexual abuse from anyone in the extended family can be overlooked as having been warranted or simply unimportant; many women may feel they deserve or have tempted the physical or sexual attack and that men have the right to beat them (Abu-Ras, 2007; Al-Krenawi et al., 2004). Women are encouraged to remain silent about rape as they can ruin their chances of marriage if no longer considered a virgin (Al-Krenawi, 2005a) or prompt the husband to seek a new, more virtuous, wife (Al-Krenawi et al., 2004). Quite often, rather than the man being prosecuted, the woman bears the brunt of the shame that still befalls the family. Despite attempts by many Muslim leaders to reinterpret or renounce such violent attitudes, some Muslim men, sometimes with the help of sympathetic mothers and other women, still carry out honor killings too often in every country (Abu-Rabia, 2011).

Divorce

Divorce is allowable, though discouraged, under Islam. It is not allowed under some orthodox Christian religions (Armstrong, 1993). Since family is sometimes the only source of stability, however, a divided family often only leaves people divided and sometimes, because of the shame it brings, alone (Abu-Ras, 2007; Al-Krenawi & Graham, 1998). Women are particularly disadvantaged in divorce and often suffer emotionally and socially as outcasts from some communities. They can display more somatization, paranoid ideation, obsessive-compulsive disorder, depression, anxiety, and psychoticism than single or married women (Al-Krenawi, 2005b). Sharia does not provide for alimony after a marriage, and a divorced woman is relegated to looking after herself or agreeing to be a second or third, often less valued, wife to another man (regardless of the law). Sharia dictates that the children belong to the father at a very young age, so the estranged wife may also lose access to her children, despite what is mandated by courts. Because divorce is not accepted in orthodox Christian relations and made so difficult overall, many wives and mothers in Arab families will endure many hardships to avoid being cast out or worse by the community (Abudabbeh, 2005; Al-Krenawi et al., 2004; Erickson & Al-Timimi, 2001).

Similar to a no-fault divorce, under Qura'nic rule, if the wife returns her dowry and pledges no claim to any of the man's property, the couple can be divorced under Sharia (Surah 4.229: Al-Hilali & Khan, 1996). This is known as *Al-Khul* (divorce). How a dowry is to be paid out may differ considerably, but in many cases, a good part of it may be put aside to be paid out to the woman in the case of a divorce. This is supposed to discourage the man rather than the woman (Fargues, 2001). However, gaining a faultless *khul*, which means giving this money back, would naturally hinder the woman's decision. This is often because of her isolation or her complete dependence upon her husband and family. It will be quite common to encounter a woman who has no idea as to her husband's finances and is in no position to support herself should anything happen. As well, there is also the problem with older women that the value of her dowry has diminished with inflation. A woman might feel it is impossible to survive without whatever her husband may mete out, and women are known to go through incredible hardship in marriage simply because they feel they have no recourse (Al-Krenawi & Graham, 1998; Yamani, 2008).

Polygamy

Perhaps a leftover from high-context traditions, polygamy is permitted for Muslim men through some interpretations of Sharia law. Though illegal even in a number of Middle East countries, practitioners may see polygamy practiced under the radar even in America; a husband and wife may divorce legally, for example, but could still remain married under Sharia law. The first wife is often relegated to a less favored position (Al-Krenawi, 2005a; Al-Krenawi, 2013). The Qur'an specifically addresses polygamy in Surah 4.2 (Al-Hilali & Khan, 1996), which is said to allow a man to marry two or three or four women (again, some interpretations are not as specific as others; see: MLibray, 2012). Surah 4.2 and Surah 4.129 (Al-Hilali & Khan, 1996) state that each wife must be treated equally and with justice by the husband. Many imams and scholars decry there is demonstrably little attention paid to these dictates, some even referring to clinical studies that find that women experience great difficulties in polygamous marriages (Al-Krenawi, 2013). Further, there is a great debate in Islam as to whether Mohammed's revelation in Surah 4.129 that "you will never be able to do perfect justice between wives even if it is your ardent desire ..." was actually, though he recognized the practice (as everyone) throughout the regions, trying to caution against the practice (Abu-Odeh, 2004; Al-Hibri, 1997).

Many men refer to Muhammad who married more than one woman after the death of his first wife with whom he had remained monogamous. Reformers, however, debate that this was more for political reasons: Surah 4.2 suggests that polygamy would be a way to treat the abandoned women of vanquished people with honor (Al-Hibri, 1997; Al-Hilali & Khan, 1996; MLibrary, 2012). Further, his last wife, Aisha, was the daughter of an ally and, since she was so young, may have been considered by Muhammad as a successor because she would mature in the ways of Islam (Armstrong, 1993; Denny, 2006; Goldschmidt & Davidson, 2006).

ARAB PEOPLE IN AMERICA

Whether newcomers or second or third generation, Arab Americans can still have strong relationships with extended families in the original homeland. The first Arab immigration between about 1880 and 1914 were mainly Christians from Syria and Lebanon escaping marginalization or persecution. Most were economically stable and eventually integrated well into the North American landscape (Abu Baker, 2003; Hodge, 2005). The second main influx occurred after the 1948 declaration of Israel and the event known as the *Nakba* where thousands of Arab people were terrorized and displaced within Israel and throughout the neighboring countries (Ghanim, 2011). These people were already traumatized by events in their homeland but relatively ignored as such in America (Al Krenawi, 2012; Gearing et al., 2013). These misplaced Arabs from Israel and surrounds were leaving some family behind and moving to a country that supported Palestinians' *oppressors*: Israel. Their ancestors still carry deep sympathies and resentments for their lost homes (Al-Krenawi, 2012; Ghanim, 2011).

The third influx of Arab people began after the Arab Israel War of 1967 and often comprised people escaping violence and brutal suppression in the name of national and sometimes religious unification in most of the 22 nations that make up the Arab League. The prevailing attitude was one of Arab nationalism against meddlesome Russian, American, and European powers seen to be supporting diverse loyalties throughout the region for their own gain rather than for what made sense locally (Erickson & Al-Timimi, 2001; Gearing et al., 2013). Many immigrants in this third wave also experienced a much cooler reception in the United States as America became far more involved in Middle Eastern affairs. Before 2001, immigrants from the third influx had already assimilated into mainstream society less and were more active in creating Muslim schools and charities and in revitalizing the language (Erickson & Al-Timimi, 2001). Many immigrants from violent backgrounds, now and in the past, have borne the scars that make fitting in troublesome: high rates of depression, anxiety, post-traumatic stress disorder, substance abuse, somatization, and other psycho-social or psychotic symptoms and psychiatric diagnoses resulting in decreased positive life and health perception (Abu Baker, 2003; Ahmed and Reddy, 2007; Al-Krenawi, 2005a; Harel-Fisch et al., 2010). While the United States generally ignored the distinguishing and traumatic reasons for immigration, in an area as diverse as the Middle East, it can be important to know why each person has had to leave home. Religious, tribal, socioeconomic, and resultant political status differences have often left a mark on an Arab immigrant's identity that may last through generations (Abu Baker, 2003; Erickson & Al-Timimi, 2001).

Stereotyping, Hatred, Acculturation, and the Struggle for Identity

Many Arab people suspect that *the West* does not care for or condone their various ways of life (Al-Krenawi, 2012; Erickson & Al-Timimi, 2001). Aside from the Arab students and professionals who may live here temporarily, there is less influx of Arab people. Erickson and Al-Timimi (2001) and Soheilian and Inman (2009) summarize the vilification of Arab and Muslim people in the press and the general media. It is a cutting negative stereotype, labeling Arabs as bloodthirsty, barbaric, hot-blooded, irrational, anti-Western, dangerous terrorists; Islam is denounced as oppressive, fundamentalist, violent, fanatical, close-minded ... the list goes on and on. As with all stereotypes, small pieces of traditions, religious doctrine, and other experience are taken out of context and pieced together as labels that aggravate the suspicions that already exist between each party.

A 2005 study showed that Arab people, especially Muslims, find acculturation within the United States more difficult than other immigrants; with increased racial marginalization, many feel they are outsiders, and many newer people especially ultimately wish to return home (Al-Krenawi & Graham, 2005, p. 301). Many fear that the vilification is for many reasons: to increase support for foreign policy in the Middle East; an inability to distinguish between those few who commit terrorist acts and the remaining population; the result of the small amount of accurate information that many Americans receive about life in the Middle East; and the still largely self-perpetuating negative images and misinformation that fills that void (Erickson & Al-Timimi, 2001; Said, 1979, 1981).

The Federal Bureau of Investigation recorded a 1,600% increase in hate crimes against Arab and Muslim people after 9/11 (Ahmed & Reddy, 2007). In just 8 months after 9/11, 30% of Arab people and 50% of Muslim people reported discrimination: Mosques and businesses owned by Arabs or Muslims were vandalized while people who even looked as if they may be Muslim or Arab were being verbally and physically assaulted or murdered (Padela & Heisler, 2010). This hatred was waged against men and women, Christians and Muslims, newcomers, second or third generations; most were married people and contributing members of society (Padela & Heisler, 2010). The Patriot Act and other bills have increased the scrutiny, arrest, incarceration, and possible deportation of Arab people throughout the United States—all of it helping to keep Arab Americans on edge (Abudabbeh, 2005; Hodge, 2005; Padela & Heisler, 2010; Soheilian & Inman, 2009).

Despite being of diverse backgrounds, many Arab Americans have been highly influenced by events in the Middles East, if not as being or knowing of victims themselves, then as the recipients of hatred from Americans despite their non-involvement (Abudabbeh, 2005). Besides the return to Islam or Christianity as a reassertion of identity (Castells, 2010), Americans have also witnessed the rejuvenation of cultural and national identities in Arab countries during the Arab Spring, the implications of which are discussed and fought not only in the Arab countries but in the American national and Arab American institutions. This has renewed some ethnic tensions throughout (Hamid, 2012; Hulett, 2011; Institute, 2012).

Despite our call for more personal freedom and women's rights, there are still very strict rules on dating and sexuality and a renewed sense of the role of religion in people's lives (Al-Krenawi & Graham, 2005). A young person who might normally rebel as part of expressing individuality (a more *Western* concept) can be seen to be questioning the cherished identity structure of the family and their entire heritage (Ahmed & Reddy, 2007). More important, increasing domestic violence is even less reported to anyone outside the family or cultural community because of the fear and mistrust of Western authorities (Abu-Ras, 2007).

Such increased distress leads to poorer mental and general health and lower levels of happiness (Amer & Harvey, 2012). There are no differences found between Christian and Muslim Arabs (Padela & Heisler, 2009, p. 287), and 48.5% of the tested population were at medium risk for experiencing an anxiety or affective disorder (Ahmed & Reddy, 2007, pp. 287–288). Such high scores normally place people in a situation whereby counseling or at least reference to self-help material is recommended; many of these people may need anti-suicidal counseling (Padela & Heisler, 2009). Such feelings of unworthiness and lack of a sense of place and security have led to many psycho-social problems such as a rise in domestic violence and the use of alcohol and drugs by Arab men in particular (Abu Bas, 2007; Al-Krenawi et al., 2004; Arfken et al., 2009; Harel-Fisch et al., 2010; Jackson & Samuels, 2011).

Those who pursue more assimilative practices feel the pressures of those who feel they should be more traditional, even while being more traditional can precipitate discriminations against their identity outside the security of their homes (Erickson & Al-Timimi, 2001). Many feel a need to internalize a number of "cultures" or identities (Arfken et al., 2009; Erikson & Al-Timimi, 2001). For example, despite general public questioning, women may be pressured to wear hijab not only by their husbands, families, and communities but by their interpretation of religion. Byng (2010) suggests the hijab may have "extended beyond the classic topics of patriarchy, Islamic feminism, religiosity, and identity to include the national identities of Western nations, the assimilation of Muslim minorities, and the potential threat of Islamic terrorism" (p. 1). Hodge (2005) continues that women may wear hijab and modest clothing as a direct repudiation of Western *immodesty* and even overtly sexual behavior (Erickson & Al-Timimi, 2001). This debate typifies internal conflicts that challenge self-identity and the meanings of *correct* behavior that can abound within especially the Arab American woman and men.

Ghaffari and Çiftçi (2009) found that increased perception of discrimination against Muslims often causes especially men to *increase* their religiosity rather than succumb to pressure. Rather than assimilate, some Arab American men decide instead to assert their traditional identities more resolutely; some even against parents who may have become more assimilated (Al-Krenawi et al., 2004, p. 109). Either way, generations of Arab Americans can be often stuck between what their parents want of them, what others in their extended communities expect of them, what they themselves want, and whether they feel accepted in society overall (Arfken et al., 2009; Ghaffari & Çiftçi, 2009; Lavalee & Poole, 2010). Various literature points out that many Arab American men and women are living between at least two cultures or identities and are thus subject to high risk of physical and mental distress (Al-Krenawi & Graham, 2005). With an understanding of the challenges Arab Americans may generally face in American society, we can now look at some more specific ideas about working with Arab American people.

Treatment of Marital and Related Problems: Culturally Sensitive Intervention

An Arab American's marriage is often much more than simply the consummation of love between two individuals. Quite the contrary, for many it is an arrangement negotiated and approved of by the family, strictly regulated by the goals and traditions of the cultural community and of faith that demand adherence. A practitioner is potentially treating a client who is torn between many viewpoints and pressures. There may be more than one community to consider: our overall community, which may too often look down on the Arab person; the closer cultural community in America that may chastise a fellow Arab for ignoring their heritage and; the community of the homeland where extended families and friends expect those in America to represent them well. We see different opinions on arranged marriages by the man, the woman, and the families. We may see problems of abuse that are justified by both the man and the wife under religious dictate. We shall see shortly that a person may also carry strict ideas of how mental illnesses that result from poor marriages and this strong identity pressure should be treated. When considering this, we shall question some of the "normal" ways in which a social worker or similar practitioner may offer or deliver services.

Many Arab Americans do not seek professional help aside from the family doctor simply because they feel most staff in such offices and facilities do not understand them (Abu-Ras, 2007; Chen & Kazanjian, 2005; Reitmanova and Gustafson, 2008). Marriage counselors, psychiatrists, social workers, financial counselors and those of the more *Western* professions may take for granted that their services are understood and desired (Al-Krenawi et al., 2004; Al-Krenawi, 2005a; Ben-Arye et al., 2009; Erickson & Al-Timimi 2001). Social workers must challenge their own viewpoints, and those of their profession, to consider exactly how well they understand and deal with Arab American concerns and how that may contrast perhaps to how the Arab American client may view the encounter (Abu-Ras, 2007).

Sorting through Differences

In this discussion, we have emphasized the layers of cultural identity in an Arab American person tempered by the variables of acculturation, education, and stereotyping that a culturally competent practitioner must consider. Such treatment must coincide with the expectations and practices of the cultural community and likely the entire family rather than the individual (Hurdle, 2002, p. 186). Effective communication becomes a key. Lu, Lum, and Chen (2001) add that a practitioner must also be critically thinking and should consider using their client as a cultural informant (Hurdle, 2002). Urban and Orbe (2010) refer to the multidimensional and holistic nature of identity in interconnected layers: personally in self-concept and definition, actively in the social practice that a person manifests, relationally in how identities are negotiated with others, and communally as the beliefs and discourse or collective memory of various communities affect the person. They also refer to identity gaps: between the sense of self and the ability to communicate this to others; between the outsider's perceptions of a person as different than that person's self-concept; and between the person's self-concept, the self the person portrays to others, and the identity that is actually seen and accepted by others (Al-Krenawi, 2012; Urban & Orbe, 2010, p. 306).

Congress (2004) uses the Culturagram as a way to assess the client's cultural contexts. In her case study of a Mexican family, Congress accounts for 10 areas of cultural identity for consideration: (1) reasons for relocation, (2) legal status, (3) time in community, (4) language spoken at home and in the community, (5) health beliefs, (6) crisis events, (7) holidays and special events, (8) contact with cultural and religious institutions, (9) values about education and work, and (10) values about family–structure, power, myths, and rules (see also Abu Baker, 2003). By *time in community*, this Culturagram implies the need to consider the degree of acculturation with the client in the new, sometimes hostile environments mentioned above. Acculturation involves "a process of adaptation and change whereby a person or an ethnic, social, religious, language, or national group integrates with or adapts to the cultural values and patterns of the majority group" (cited in Al-Krenawi & Graham, 2005, pp. 310–311). However, we should remember that time in community will not necessarily mean that a person has accepted local thought, especially when there is revival of more traditional concepts of marriage and gender. We will consider what effect essentializing or stereotyping has on a client's need, desire, or capacity for acculturation, as well as to what degree the society and social worker are willing to adapt to the client (Abu Baker, 2003; Al-Krenawi & Graham, 2005; Kumar, Seay, & Karabenick, 2011). The practitioner must resist two temptations: first, to jump to any conclusion as to which specific aspect of a person's cultural and personal background is more germane to their self-identity and, second, that a person is in fact interested in acculturating into the American community, particularly as many may only be here temporarily for scholastic or professional engagements (Urban & Orbe, 2010).

Honor and Stigma

We must emphasize the potential problems encountered by a client in maintaining honor in their community and being shunned. Practitioners may see people ostracized sometimes because of their

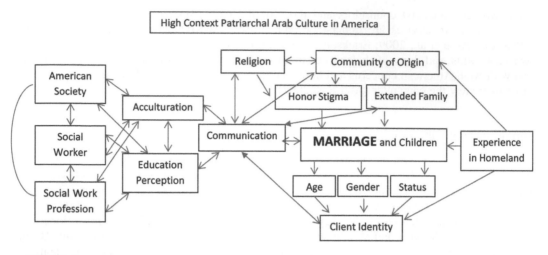

FIGURE 1   Interrelationship between marriage and family and social workers, where communication is the center.

perceived *indiscretions*. The concept of honor and shunning sin (such as in drinking, gambling, and sexual indiscretion) is mentioned in the Qur'an as in the Bible (for example, Surahs 4.31, 42.37, 74.5, and 5.90 in MLlibray, 2012). We have also mentioned that the honor of a man is found in his ability to keep his wife and family free from sin and dishonor. The ability to maintain a good marriage in the eyes of a high-context community is essential to maintaining a sense of honor for the bride, the groom, and their families. It may be imperative that silence be kept over difficulties the couple may be having. For example, a person seeking help for mental health issues may be branded *majnun* (pronounced "muhj-noon") or crazy, a term that carries considerable stigma as it implies a spiritual illness (Abudabbeh, 2005; Erickson & Al-Timimi, 2001). Despite local laws, simply a person with marital problems and illness can be isolated from the community; a woman further removed for example by being forced to drop work or studies or other contact with the public (Al-Krenawi et al., 2004). Men gain an excuse to remarry; to find a better wife, perhaps to have *better* children (Al-Krenawi et al., 2004; Cross & Bloomer, 2010). We can understand why a client may be initially unwilling to discuss problems.

Figure 1 helps to pull the discussion together. In it, we see the relationship between religion and the community of origin or cultural likeness and how they form the top of the hierarchy. Marriage and children are roughly at the center of society with influence filtering down from religion and community tempered by honor and stigma that motivates much of the family's practice. The identity of the client is, in turn, tempered by gender, age, and status both within the family and within the community.

Religion

Several studies suggest that still not enough is done to assess the effectiveness of faith-based social services (Boddie & Cnann, 2006; Fischer & Stelter, 2006). "It should be noted that faith-based providers are closer to the recipients of the services than are public civil servants and therefore tend to have better information about local needs" (Boddie & Cnaan, 2006, p. 288). Abu-Ras (2007) suggests that the American practitioner must consider faith-based diagnoses and treatment; similar efforts are being made for other cultural groups (Abu-Ras, 2007; Boddie & Cnaan, 2006; Lavallie & Poole, 2010). Practitioners must accept that religious practice may provide the soothing that replaces the need for drugs or similar (Boddie & Cnaan, 2006; Ghaffari & Çiftçi, 2009). With lack of proper understanding of faith and perception, there are real fears of misdiagnosis and mistreatment (Abudabbeh, 2005; Al-Krenawi, 2005b; Al-Krenawi & Graham, 2006; Cross and Bloomer, 2010; Ferguson, 2004; Gearing et al., 2013). Cross and Bloomer (2010) quote two very important questions raised by Kleinman: "To what extent do psychiatric disorders differ in different societies [and] ... Does the standard approach to cross-cultural research in psychiatry commit a 'category fallacy' (presupposing that *Western* diagnostic categories are culture-free entities)?" (p. 269).

Skinner (2010) and Sayed (2003) note the difference between a Muslim's more holistic sense of well-being and the *Westerner's* more individualistic split between the mind and the spirit. This split is seen somewhat more in Christian Arab people and, indeed, "religiosity within a Judeo-Christian context has been demonstrated to be conducive to better mental health" (Al-Krenawi et al., 2004, p. 109). This might be attributed more to the specific nature of Islamic doctrine itself, a greater reluctance to interpret and accept individual interpretations, rather than to the better acculturation of Christian Arab people. Both Christian and Muslim, however, consider very seriously spiritual ideas about meaning and purpose in life related to the supernatural world, divinities, angels and evil spirits, and otherwise. It is often for an elder of the community, most often a spiritual leader and not a social worker or doctor, to interpret the dictates of the religion, the community and the tribe. Many Arab people believe that strife is a religious punishment for some reason or the result of evil spirits having inhabited a person for wrongful acts of some kind (Cross and Bloomer, 2010). In Muslim cultures, men are inflicted by the will of God (*Insha'Allah*), and women may be possessed by evil *jinns* (spirits). Both religions can view schizophrenia, depression, and anxiety as the result of religious failings; the longing for religious fulfillment, or protection. In many Arab societies, there is a prevalence of belief in sorcery (specifically outlawed in some Arab countries) and the devil, evil eye (Al-Krenawi et al., 2004; Hodge, 2004; Sayed, 2003).

The Qur'an in particular documents coping and healing mechanisms for marital problems and for illnesses, such as increased prayer and practice of the other Pillars of Islam. These may actually work for many problems that Muslims might experience (Boddie & Cnaan, 2006; Denny, 2006; Ghaffari & Çiftçi, 2009). Despite more *Westernized* education and changing attitudes, surprisingly high numbers of Arab people in the Middle East (up to 85% of young Arab women in one study) still use prayer as a part of overall therapy (Al-Krenawi et al., 2004; Abdel-Khalek, 2010). Erickson and Al-Timimi (2001) argue that many Arab people are less conditioned to consider things *psychologically* and thus do not spend time in self-analysis and prescription. Abdulrahim and Ajrouch (2010) describe in detail a client who "did not invoke any particular health-related criteria. Instead he saw [his poor] health as being wholly integrated within the social context in which he lived, and his inability to achieve balance or live in harmony" (p. 1236). It is typical that "didactic and structured therapies are more easily adjusted to or accepted by Arab American clients than in-depth or insight-oriented therapies" (Al-Krenawi, 2005b, p. 564). Cross and Bloomer (2010) note importantly that "Models of causality are now including epistemological and ontological paradigms, which interact to identify mental illness across many cultures" (p. 269).

Marriage Problems in the Family and the Community Environment

The practitioner may find it very difficult to conduct confidential interviews as the family often remain arbiters in what is said and in forms of treatment (Sayed, 2003; Srour, 2005). Though more Arab American women pursue careers in America, many may still be considered subservient to or suppressed by paternalistic attitudes. Many wives will still defer to their husbands for all major family decisions (Al-Krenawi & Graham, 2006). Women will often be accompanied to the practitioner's office. With men and women, the acceptance of the diagnosis, treatment, and need for follow-up may revert back to the family and community who may decide whether treatment is complete or lacking. Further treatment may be referred back to avenues within the honored traditional community (Al-Krenawi et al., 2004; Erickson & Al-Timimi, 2001; Ferguson, 2005; Sayed, 2003).

We must remember how the status of a person can change with deviances from community expectations. Problems especially within new Arab American families are often seen with the loss of the extended family support (Ahmed & Reddy, 2007), and extreme loneliness can set in especially where a family does not yet feel accepted overall (Abu Baker, 2006). This sense of status may carry over from the homeland, which can affect a man or woman when, for example, a person who had status and leadership roles in their old home may now have to marry beneath his or her previous station or simply defer his or her higher position and influence to others (Abu Baker, 2006).

Men can become more philandering in the more liberal environment or violent in their inability to control their family. The prominence of heavy-handed patriarchy in many Arab families is extended to the oldest son or extended family male in the absence of the father (Abudabbeh, 2005; Al-Krenawi, 2013; Al-Krenawi & Graham, 2005). Studies show how such stressors mentioned above seem to build up within married women. Women's isolation and depression can increase within bad marriages that afford them little respect or recourse to assistance. Yet, voicing that distress and concern may only lead to further dismissal or marginalization within the entire extended family and the community (Al-Krenawi et al., 2004).

There are many stressors on a marriage. Norris, Arolin, and Nickerson (2011) document the great sense of loss that many immigrants or refugees have from being forced to move from their home, suggesting further that a practitioner should include a screening for such grief at the beginning of sessions. There are many frustrating things that an Arab person may have to deal with in America: basic things, for example, like where a Muslim person might find a bank that follows Islamic Sharia ideas on matters of interest. Many Muslims must adapt their diet due to a relative lack of *halal* foods at times (similar to a Jewish person's requirements for kosher foods). Parents and elders may feel inadequate when their children who are more adept with English and new systems must guide them through social situations. People feel shame when they are forced to take lesser jobs, often because their education, qualifications, and work history are either poorly documented or not accepted (Abu Baker, 2006; Arfken et al., 2009). We have mentioned that Arab American Muslims may still prefer to seek help from traditional healers, religious leaders such as the Imam in the mosque who understand them and meet their expectations and recognize spiritual and community elements in their treatment (Cross & Bloomer, 2010; Sayed, 2003; Skinner, 2010). Cross and Bloomer say that these "concerns might not be shared with the clinician unless a trusting relationship is established" (p. 270). We see the need for both much further education and partnerships with the community and spiritual help groups (Ben Ayre et al., 2009; Ferguson, 2004).

Practitioners are challenged when their profession promotes the quick removal of children and women from violent, abusive, or criminal situations. Social services intended to help people in domestic abuse can be the least utilized of all by Arab Americans. Victims tend to resort first to legal, family, and simple medical services (Abu-Ras, 2007). However, "mediators within the community may be approached to help social workers or other professionals work with families to reconcile differences and facilitate compromise, while allowing each party within the family to save face by not 'giving in'" (Al-Krenawi & Graham, 2005, p. 302). Individuation is not immediately advisable, and removal of people from the home for example may be almost as harmful to the person's well-being as the original problem. (Erickson & Al-Timimi, 2001). The cultural community is where crucial information against domestic violence, problems with drugs, and other such social problems can be disseminated (Abu-Ras, 2007; Elsaidi, 2011). Most criminal justice and similar interventions should be seen to be complementary to the community's efforts.

This practice also helps to give the practitioner credibility within the cultural community (Al-Krenawi et al., 2004; Al-Krenawi, 2013; Ferguson, 2005; Gearing et al., 2013; Harel-Fisch et al., 2010; Soheilian & Inman, 2009).

Rather than being considered simply the source of stigma to a family, the community should be considered a resource (Hodge, 2005). Community leaders know the prejudice and stereotyping that may follow an Arab person: They know the individual and likely of the traumas and distress emanating from experiences in their homeland or in their new environment (Erickson & Al-Timimi, 2001; Lavallie & Poole, 2010). The community can mediate in generational clashes or problems with acculturation (Al-Krenawi, 2005b; Ferguson, 2005; Al-Krenawi & Graham, 2006; Abu Baker, 2006; Bodie & Cnaan, 2006). Cross and Bloomer (2010) continue to say that "... because the clinician had engaged in culturally responsive interactions ... demonstrating knowledge of culture and ethnicity, as well as contextualizing the client's problems, the clinician was seen as more credible" (p. 275).

Abu-Ras (2007) suggests that women are just as afraid that men who have trouble with the law will be deported. Indeed, Abu Baker (2006) extends this to new Arab people in general, whose legal status may still be in flux and, with the increasingly negative stereotyping, thus feel authorities will not understand or treat their problems properly.

Sexuality and Marriage

Social workers must understand the problem that many Arab Americans may have with discussing sexuality—generally more easily and liberally expressed and practiced in America than in the Middle East. Many women can be quickly accused of being too promiscuous, defined very conservatively in comparison to many more liberal American definitions, or for courting without permission or accompaniment.

Problems in sexuality and sexual practice may be solved with careful negotiation and compromise; referring to the honor of the family can still help a practitioner gain entry. Considering how some sexual virtue is directly mentioned in the Qur'an, though difficult, simply understanding that these affairs must be negotiated in a quiet way, with the right people involved, may help. How men and women treat one another can be directly related to how important it is to have children, especially sons to carry the family name. In fact, the practitioner must consider how the aforementioned concerns, virtue, honor, piety, punishment, alcohol abuse, guilt, loss of family control, and duality of identity can enter easily into the development of poor marital relationships without a word being spoken to the practitioner *outside* the family.

Both men and women will be chastised for espousing homosexuality or other sexual preference (Abudabbeh, 2005; Al-Krenawi & Graham, 2006). However, some studies have shown that a shared concern about homosexuality among Arab men was actually that it precluded procreation and thus the strong heritage lines, especially in new countries (Hooghe, Dejaeghere, Claes, & Quintelier, 2010). Despite religious condemnation, there may be quiet negotiated tolerance for homosexual behavior that does not interfere with the family's honor; that translates sometimes as being married and procreating regardless of extra-marital activities (Bradley, 2010; Hooge et al., 2008/2010). As well, it is not unheard of to hire surrogates to either impregnate a woman or to give birth to a child when one or the other is sterile (Zeitzen, 2008).

Isolation and Confidentiality

Abudabbeh (2005) suggests that some Arab American women find it easier to phone for assistance from practitioners, especially when anonymity is at stake. This can also help women who are simply less mobile or those who are concerned about their situation but afraid others may learn of their seeking help. Studies of Arab women seeking help indicate that medical general practitioners, rather than psychologists, psychiatrists, or other mental health professionals, tend to be the targeted treatment source of choice (Al-Krenawi & Graham, 2005). Perhaps this is also because it may be easier to hide the cost of a visit to the doctor as a general consultation rather than the expense of visiting another professional (Abu-Ras, 2007). For all such reasons, Al-Krenawi et al. (2004) recommend placing social service consultations and mental health clinics within the framework of less stigmatizing general health clinics.

It is difficult to keep people out of the communication circle. "The cultural context in which treatment occurs is patriarchal; rather than challenging these cultural structures carte blanche, the treatment emphasizes empowering women and men within existing power relations ..." (Al-Krenawi & Graham, 2005, p. 301). Men might often need to be cajoled to attend therapy sessions, especially for themselves. However, this is more easily accomplished when a practitioner might ask them to attend ostensibly to be consulted about women or children under their domain. Regardless, men, whether they wish to attend or do not, must generally be included in the treatment scenario under some guise.

Confidentiality is considered differently in many Arab environments, and some husbands, for example, may consider it their right to hear all personal details of his family's problems. Clients who receive constant reassurance that their confidence is kept wherever possible may soon become more compliant. As well, Cross and Bloomer (2010) suggests that a client and practitioner should cooperate and collude more on diagnosis and treatment to achieve better communication and compliance.

Communication, Linguistics, and the Chain of Discussion

Frequent and effective communication is a key to successful understanding between all parties: the social worker, American society that can often dictate the profession, the Arab American communities, the families, and the individuals. Since this is a two-way street, the degree to which this communication is successful will depend on each person's level of education as opposed to stereotypical perceptions and the degree of acculturation in all parties. Second, there are, as we shall explore, various ways of communicating or demonstrating marital problems and symptoms of illness. The practitioner must consider not only different ways that psycho-social problems may be understood and communicated but, likely through communication with many new sources, alternative ways to diagnose and treat them.

Second- or third-generation Arab Americans may certainly be more fluent in English, but there may still be linguistics nuances they have adopted from their heritage. Consider, for example, how language is used in tandem with body language and in the context of cultural habits or understandings. Arabic-speaking practitioners, just as English-speaking Arab Americans, may find the use of certain phrases or other communication techniques cryptic. These might include somatization of mental health issues, the use of proverbs by many Arab people to describe certain ideas, and a tendency to underemphasize the severity or prevalence of symptomology when describing their problem. After conquering all previous challenges, misdiagnosis can still occur here (Cross & Bloomer, 2010).

One study of Egyptian men, for example, found that many expressed depression and anxiety through agitation, somatic symptoms, and the translation of feeling into body language rather than as vocalized ideas of guilt, sin, and reproach we might find in more *Western* cultures (Al-Krenawi, 2005b). Many Muslim women and men feel obliged by Islamic dictates to refrain from eye contact with the opposite sex when they are not related; we may consider such body language a sign of resistance to treatment but women especially may simply be exercising their discretion (Al-Krenawi, 2005b). Finally, Al-Krenawi (2000) suggests that Arab people explain feelings through the use of a cache of stories: a wealth of established and authoritative expressions, proverbs, poems, and metaphors that are used within a known context. Relating these proverbs and metaphors should preclude the necessity for delving into long personal explorations and reveal immediately what a person thinks, the distress or other problem they may be experiencing, in a way that is both indirect (avoiding unwanted individuation) and yet, when properly understood, concise (Al-Krenawi, 2000).

The phenomenon of somatization "... is one of the foremost reasons for the 'first filter' challenges of mental health professionals ..." (Al-Krenawi, 2005a, p. 560). Somatization is a less abstract way to deal with problems that are not as well understood in Arab cultures as they may be in more *Western* cultures (Abu-Ras, 2007; Erickson & Al-Timimi, 2001). Sayed (2003) reminds us of the ways in which Western people can also use somatization when they refer to *having a broken heart* or to *having the gall* to do something. A good understanding of these idioms provides even more lucid ideas of how a patient is actually being effected, and provide language with which the practitioner can begin to connect with the client and assist (Al-Krenawi et al., 2004).

Communication can be very cyclical. Practitioners may find that authoritarian families have a triangular type of consultation: the mother who cares for the children may know more about a child's problems and so must advise the father, who would be involved with the practitioner on what decisions are to be made. Similarly, the father may see a child as simply acting out or demonstrating a simple behavioral problem but consult with the mother as to what the problem is. A practitioner may find the same cyclical or indirect communication, consulting with other family or community members, effective or necessary as well when attempting to gain information or gain compliance from a client (Al-Krenawi et al., 2004).

Such circular communication also arises from client understanding that speaking out against other family members is often irreparably damaging, especially of course with family members present (Dwairy, 2006). Such talk *spreads the pain*, which many clients do not wish to do (Abudabbeh, 2005; Al-Krenawi & Graham, 2006; Srour, 2005). As well, direct or open discussion can be considered rude, and any sign of anger or frustration is looked down upon. This further impairs the ability of a practitioner to gain intimacy within the family. Where more *Western* families may benefit from knowing how they are perceived within the family and work to understand one another's motivations and fears, the desire for such knowledge may be more limited within traditional Arab families. Thus, much can remain unsaid (Abudabbeh, 2005; Dwairy, 2006). Sometimes, again, the only recourse is to attempt to gain information and compliance through indirect sources such as the cultural community who often know their constituents well.

Practitioners should also consider their own method of asking questions or delivering verdicts, diagnoses, prescriptions, and other statements to Arab American clients. It may be futile to try to force clinical realities upon a person (Hurdle, 2002; Sayed, 2003). An Arab American's sense of time may be somewhat different than another American; since many things happen by the will of God (*Insha'Allah* for Muslim people); time is not pressing. To ask such a client to consider the hypothetical consequences of decisions, or to predict the future of certain treatments, can be ineffective as the client may simply consider this strange and unreasonable (Erickson & Al-Timimi, 2001).

Besides community leaders, cultural mediators may be used to bridge these gaps (Al-Krenawi & Graham, 2001; Cross & Bloomer, 2010). Sayed (2003) mentions that interpreters can become caught up in the problem experienced by the original patient. Should a patient be working on particularly difficult problems, the interpreter may start to experience feelings of depression or similar because of the bad nature of the problem. However, it can be very beneficial to have a true mediator who can interpret not just the linguistic traditions above but, like community members, can share with the social worker many of the ideas and conventions, or challenges, faced by Arab Americans of so many different backgrounds (Al-Krenawi & Graham, 2001).

Acquiescence and Compliance

Since social workers are revered as *experts*, the client may simply acquiesce in the practitioner's expertise. A client who does not understand the purpose of social workers, psychologists, and other helping practitioners may treat the practitioner as simply a medical doctor for strictly biological medical issues. Clients, and their chaperones, expect simple detailed advice, explicit directions, and medication. This may actually prove more productive in the short term than intricate self-searching and self-assessing practice. Erickson and Al-Timimi (2001) suggest that it may be advisable to avoid or at least couch certain clinical terms in other language—especially those clinical designations and prescriptions that may be considered denigrating, marginalizing, and stigmatizing (see also Hurdle, 2002).

The client will likely only work on solutions that make sense not only for the client (Al-Krenawi & Graham, 2006; Al-Krenawi et al., 2004; Ferguson, 2005; Sayed, 2003; Srour, 2004). The practitioner will have to carefully monitor outcomes to ensure success and to possibly circumvent misunderstandings or misdiagnoses of why a client may have strayed from prescribed treatments and plans (Ferguson, 2005; Sayed, 2003). When working with clients from Arab background, social worker are encouraged to set up achievable goals in the first or second session. The fact that some or all of these goals can be achieved successfully will contribute significantly to build trust and good working alliances with clients.

SUMMARY

In conclusion, it should be clear that careful consideration must be given to the complex motivations and belief structures behind Arab Americans' activities and problems they may be experiencing. It is unfair to stereotype an Arab American identity: they are far too diverse a people. Islam and Christianity are vastly shaded with a multitude of understandings and interpretations: few coming from a malicious or violent beginning. Marriage and family ae extremely important to many people, not simply to an Arab American person. However, with the added pressures from a perceived hostile public, there is a greater need for the securities and support that can only be found in traditional marriage.

Many Arab American people come from a tumultuous heritage. Whether first or second or further generation in America, their ancestors may have had to deal with troubling times that brought them first to America. Again, with growing waves of mistrust in the United States, some have returned to strong religiosity as a form of identity and comfort, while others may have never left it. This is not a violent retaliation; it is a reaffirmation of the entities they hope to trust.

However, it is not enough even to understand these motivations. Social workers must be flexible in their practice to accommodate some of these beliefs. As well, there are still the nuances of linguistics and social experience that will shade a person's desire to consult with social workers and similar practitioners and understand the consultation. Communication is the key to working with people within their very influential cultural community: the community that helps the social worker to appreciate the beliefs and needs, and can disseminate instructive words and advise toward maintaining better health care throughout the community. Trust is an essential element, and it comes and is maintained through serious study, understanding, negotiation, and action among all parties.

REFERENCES

Abdel-Khalek, A. M. (2010). Religiosity, subjective well-being, and neuroticism. *Mental Health, Religion & Culture*, *13*(1), 67–79.

Abdulrahim, S., & Ajrouch, K. (2010). Social and cultural meanings of self-rated health: Arab immigrants in the United States. *Qualitative Health Research, 20*(9), 1229–1240.

Abu Baker, K. (2003). Marital problems among Arab families: Between cultural and family therapy. *Arab Studies Quarterly, 25*(4), 53–74.

Abudabbeh, N. (2005). Arab families. In M. McGoldrick, J. Giordano, & M. Garcia-Preto (Eds.), *Ethnicity and family therapy* (pp. 423–436). New York, NY: Guildford Press.

Abu-Odeh, L. (2004). Egyptian feminism: Trapped in the identity debate. In Y. Y. Haddad, & B. F. Stowasser (Eds.), *Islamic law and the challenges of modernity* (pp. 183–212). Walnut Creek, CA: Altamira Books.

Abu-Rabia, A. (2011). Family honor killings: Between custom and state law. *The Open Psychology Journal, 4*(Suppl 1-M4), 34–44.

Abu-Ras, W. (2007). Cultural beliefs and service utilization by battered Arab immigrant women. *Violence against women, 13*(10), 1002–1025.

Ahmed, S., & Reddy, L. A. (2007). Understanding the mental health needs of American Muslims: Recommendations and considerations for practice. *Journal of Multicultural Counseling and Development, 35*, 207–216.

Al-Hibri, A. (1997). Islam, law, and custom: Redefining Muslim women's rights. *American University International Law Review, 12*(1), 1–44.

Al-Hilali, M. T., & Khan, M. M. (1996). *The noble Qur'an: Translations of the meanings in the English language.* Madinah: King Fahd Complex for the Printing of the Holy Qur'an.

Al-Krenawi, A. (2000). Bedouin-Arab clients' use of proverbs in the therapeutic setting. *International Journal for the Advancement of Counselling, 22*, 91–102.

Al-Krenawi, A. (2005a). Islam, human rights and social work in a changing world. Paper presented at University of Calgary, Canada.

Al-Krenawi, A. (2005b). Mental health practice in Arab countries. *Current Opinion in Psychiatry, 18*(5), 560–564.

Al-Krenawi, A. (2012). *Tomorrow's players: The Israeli-Palestinian case.* New York, NY: Nova publisher.

Al-Krenawi, A. (2013). Mental health and polygamy: The Syrian case. *World Journal of Psychiatry, 22*(3), 1–7.

Al-Krenawi, A., & Graham, J. R. (1998). Divorce among Muslim Arab women in Israel. *Journal of Divorce and Remarraige, 29*(3/4), 103–119.

Al-Krenawi, A., & Graham, J. R. (2000). Culturally sensitive social work practice with Arab clients in mental health settings. *Health & Social Work, 25*(1), 9–22.

Al-Krenawi, A., & Graham, J. (2001). The cultural mediator: Bridging the gap between a non-Western community and professional social work practice. *British Journal of Social Work, 31*, 665–685.

Al-Krenawi, A., & Graham, J. R. (2003). Introduction. In A. Al-Krenawi & J. R. Graham (Ed.), *Multicultural social work in Canada: Working with diverse ethno-racial communities.* Toronto: Oxford University Press.

Al-Krenawi, A., & Graham, J. R. (2005). Marital therapy for Arab Muslim Palestinian couples in the context of reacculturation. *The Family Journal, 13*, 300–310.

Al-Krenawi, A., & Graham, J. R. (2006). A comparative study of family functioning, health, and mental health awareness and utilization among female Bedouin-Arabs from recognized and unrecognized villages in the Negev. *Health Care for Women International, 27*(2), 182–196.

Al-Krenawi, A., Graham, J. R., Dean, Y. Z., & Eltaiba, N. (2004). Cross-national study of attitudes towards seeking professional help: Jordan, United Arab Emirates (UAE) and Arabs in Israel. *International Journal of Social Psychiatry, 50*(2), 102–114.

Amer, M. M., & Hovey, J. D. (2012). Anxiety and depression in a post-September 11 sample of Arabs in the USA. *Social Psychiatry and Psychiatric Epidemiology, 47*, 409–418.

Appadurai, A. (2006). *Fear of small numbers: An essay on the geography of anger.* Durham, NC: Duke University Press.

Arab American Association. (n.d.). Arab Americans demographics. Retrieved from http://www.arabamerica.com

Arfken, C. L., Kubiak, S. P., & Farrag, M. (2009). Acculturation and polysubstance abuse in Arab-American treatment clients. *Transcultural Psychiatry, 46*(4), 608–622. doi: 10.1177/1363461509351364

Arfken, C. L., Kubiak, S. P., & Koch, A. L. (2007). Arab Americans in publicly financed substance abuse treatment. *Ethnicity & Disease, 17*, 72–76.

Armstrong, K. (1993). *A history of God: The 4,000-year quest of Judaism, Christianity, and Islam.* New York, NY: Alfred A. Knopf.

Baker, R. W. (2010). The Islamic awakening. In D. S. Sorenson (Ed.), *Interpreting the Middle East: Essential themes* (pp. 249–274). Boulder, CO: Westview Press.

Ben-Arye, E., Karkabi, K., Karkabi, S., Keshet, Y., Haddad, M., & Frenkel, M. (2009). Attitudes of Arab and Jewish patients toward integration of complementary medicine in primary care clinics in Israel: A cross-cultural study. *Social Science & Medicine, 68*(1), 177–182.

Boddie, S. C., & Cnaan, R. A. (2006). Concluding remarks. *Journal of Religion & Spirituality in Social Work: Social Thought, 25*(3–4), 287–291.

Boyle, D. P., & Springer, A. (2001). Toward a cultural competence measure for social work with specific populations. *Journal of Ethnic and Cultural Diversity in Social Work, 9*(3-4), 53–71.

Bradley, J. R. (2010). *Behind the veil of vice: The business and culture of sex and vice in the Middle East.* New York, NY: Palgrave Macmillan.

Byng, M. D. (2010). Symbolically Muslim: Media, hijab, and the West. *Critical Sociology, 36*(1), 109–129.

Castells, M. (2010). *The Power of identity* (2nd ed.). Chichester, West Sussex, United Kingdom: John Wiley & Sons, Ltd.

Chen, A. W., & Kazanjian, A. (2005). Rate of mental health service utilization by Chinese immigrants in British Columbia. *Canadian Journal of Public Health, 96*(1), 49–51.

Congress, E. P. (2004). Cultural and Ethical Issues in working with culturally diverse patients and their families: The use of the Culturagram to promote cultural competent practice in health care settings. *Social Work in Health Care, 39*(3/4), 249–262.

Cross, W. M., & Bloomer, M. J. (2010). Extending boundaries: Clinical communication with culturally and linguistically diverse mental health clients and careers. *International Journal of Mental Health Nursing, 19,* 268–277. doi: 10.1111/j.1447-0349.2010.00667

Denny, F. M. (2006). *An introduction to Islam.* Upper Saddle River, NJ: Pearson: Prentice Hall.

Dwairy, M., Achoui, M., Abouserie, R., Farah, A., Sakhleh, A. A., Fayed, M., & Khan, H. K. (2006). Parenting styles in Arab societies: A first cross-regional research study. *Journal of Cross-Cultural Psychology, 37,* 230–247.

Elsaidi, M. H. (2011). Human rights and Islamic law: A legal analysis challenging the husband's authority to punish "rebellious" wives. *Muslim Journal of Human Rights, 7*(2), 1–25.

Erickson, C. D., & Al-Timimi, N. R. (2001). Providing mental health services to Arab Americans: Recommendations and considerations. *Cultural Diversity and Ethnic Minority Psychology, 7*(4), 308–327.

Fargues, P. (2001). The new Arab family. In N. S. Hopkins (Ed.), *Cairo papers in social sciences* (vol. 24, pp. 247–273). Cairo, Egypt: The American University in Cairo Press.

Ferguson, C. J. (2004). Arab Americans: Acculturation and prejudice in an era of international conflict. In C. Negy (Ed.), *Cross-cultural psychotherapy: Toward a critical understanding of diverse clients* (pp. 265–278). Reno, NV: Bent Tree Press.

Fischer, R. L., & Stelter, J. D. (2006). Testing faith. *Journal of Religion & Spirituality in Social Work: Social Thought, 25*(3–4), 105–122.

Gearing, R. E., Schwalbe, C. S., MacKenzie, M. J., Brewer, K. B., Ibrahim, R. W., Olimat, H. S., ... Al-Krenawi, A. (2013). Adaptation and translation of mental health interventions in Middle Eastern Arabic countries: A systematic review of barriers to and strategies for effective treatment implementation. *International Journal of Social Psychiatry, 59*(7), 671–681.

Geertz, C. (2009). From the native's point of view: On the nature of anthropological understanding. In R. S. Khalef & S. Khalef (Eds.), *Arab society and culture. An essential reader* (pp. 31–41). London, UK: SAQI.

Ghaffari, A., & Çiftçi, A. (2009). Religiosity and self-esteem of Muslim immigrants to the United States: The moderating role of perceived discrimination. *International Journal for the Psychology of Religion, 20*(1), 14–25.

Ghanim, H. (2011). The Nakba. In N. N. Rouhana & A. Sabbagh-Khoury (Eds.), *The Palestinians in Israel: Readings in history, politics and society* (pp. 16–25). Mada al-Carmel, Israel: Arab Center for Applied Social Research.

Goldschmidt, A., & Davidson, L. (2006). *A concise history of the Middle East* (8th ed.). Boulder, CO: Westview Press.

Hamid, S. (2012, October 15). *Don't give up on the Arab Spring.* Retrieved from Foreign Policy: http://www.foreign policy.com/articles/2012/09/12/dont_give_up_on_the_arab_spring

Harel-Fisch, Y., Radwan, Q., Walsh, S. D., Laufer, A., Amitai, G., Fogel-Grinvald, H. ... Abdeen, Z. (2010). Psychosocial outcomes related to subjective threat from armed conflict events (STACE): Findings from the Israeli-Palestinian cross-cultural HBSC study. *Child Abuse & Neglect, 34,* 623–638.

Hodge, D. R. (2005). Social work and the house of Islam: Orienting practitioners to the beliefs and values of Muslims in the United States. *Social Work, 50*(2), 163–173.

Hoodfar, H. (2009). Marriage, family, and household in Cairo. In S. Saad Khalaf & R. Saad Khalaf (Eds.), *Arab society and culture. An essential reader* (pp. 262–277). London: SAQI.

Hooghe, M. D., Dejaeghere, Y., Claes, E., & Quintelier, E. (2010). "Yes, but suppose everyone turned gay?" The structure of attitudes toward gay and lesbian rights among Islamic youth in Belgium. *Journal of LGBT Youth, 7*(1), 49–71.

Hulett, S. (2011, October 7). *Metro Detroit Arab Americans reflect on Arab Spring, foreign policy.* Retrieved from Michigan radio: News for Michigan: http://michiganradio.org/post/metro-detroit-arab-americans-reflect-arab-spring-foreign-policy

Hurdle, D. E. (2002). Native Hawaiian traditional healing: Culturally based interventions for social work practice. *Social Work, 47*(2), 183–192.

Indian Health Service, U. D. (2009). *Indian health service trends in Indian health 2002–2003 edition.* Washington, DC: U.S. Department of Health and Human Services.

Institute, B. (2012, October 8). *Americans on the Middle East: A study of American public opinion.* Retrieved from http://www.brookings.edu/research/reports/2012/10/08-americans-middle-east-telhami

54

Jackson, K. F., & Samuels, G. M. (2011). Multiracial competence in social work: Recommendations for culturally attuned work with multiracial people. *Social Work, 56*(3), 235–245.

Kayyali, R. A. (2006). *The Arab Americans.* Westport, CT: Greenwood Press.

Kumar, R., Seay, N., & Karabenick, S. (2011). Shades of white: Identity status, stereotypes, prejudice, and xenophobia. *Educational Studies, 47,* 347–378.

Kuran, T. (2012). The economic roots of political underdevelopment in the Middle East: A historical perspective. *Southern Economic Journal, 78*(4), 1086–1095.

Lavallee, L. F., & Poole, J. M. (2010). Beyond recovery: Colonization, health and healing for indigenous people in Canada. *International Journal of Mental Health Addiction, 8,* 271–281.

Lu, Y. E., Lum, D., & Chen, S. (2001). Cultural competency and achieving styles in clinical social work. *Journal of Ethnic and Cultural Diversity in Social Work, 9*(3–4), 1–32.

Mahmood, S. (2005). *The politics of piety: The Islamic revival and the feminist subject.* Princeton, NJ: Princeton University Press.

MLibrary. (2012). *The Koran.* Retrieved from University of Michigan Online Texts: http://quod.lib.umich.edu/k/koran

National Association of Social Workers. (2008). *Code of ethics.* Retrieved from http://www.socialworkers.org/pubs/code/code.asp

Norris, A. E., Aroian, K. J., & Nickerson, D. M. (2011). Premigration persecution, postmigration stressors and resources, and postmigration mental health: A study of severely traumatized U.S. Arab immigrant women. *Journal of the American Psychiatric Nurses Association, 17*(4), 283–293.

Padela, A. I., & Heisler, M. (2010). The association of perceived abuse and discrimination after September 11, 2001, with psychological distress, level of happiness, and health status among Arab Americans. *American Journal of Public Health, 100*(2), 284–291. doi: 10.2105/AJPH.2009.164954

Reitmanova, S., & Gustafson, D. L. (2008). "They can't understand it": Maternity health and care needs of immigrant Muslim women in St. John's, Newfoundland. *Maternal Child Health Journal, 12,* 101–111.

Sabry, T. (2010). *Cultural encounters in the Arab world: On media, the modern and the everyday.* London, UK: I. B. Tauris & Co Ltd.

Said, E. (1979). *Orientalism.* New York, NY: Random House.

Said, E. (1981). *Covering Islam: How the media and the experts determine how we see the rest of the world.* New York, NY: Pantheon Books.

Sayed, M. A. (2003). Conceptualization of mental health illness within Arab cultures: Meeting challenges in cross-cultural settings. *Social Behaviour and Personality, 31*(4), 333–342.

Sidani, Y. M., & Thornberry, J. (2009). The current Arab work ethic: Antecedents, implications, and potential remedies. *Journal of Business Ethics, 91,* 35–49.

Skinner, R. (2010). An Islamic approach to psychology and mental health. *Mental Health, Religion & Culture, 13*(6), 547–551.

Soheilian, S. S., & Inman, A. G. (2009). Middle Eastern Americans: The effects of stigma on attitudes toward counseling. *Journal of Muslim Mental Health, 4*(2), 139–158.

Srour, R. W. (2005). Children living under a multi-traumatic environment: The Palestinian case. *Israeli Journal of Psychiatry Related Science, 42*(2), 88–95.

Urban, E. L., & Orbe, M. P. (2010). Identity gaps of contemporary U.S. immigrants: Acknowledging divergent communicative experiences. *Communication Studies, 61,* 304–320.

White House Commission on Complementary and Alternative Medicine Commission. (2002). White House Commission on Complementary and Alternative Medicine Policy. Retrieved from http://www.whccamp.hhs.gov/tc.html

Yamani, M. A. (2008). *Polygamy and law in contemporary Saudi Arabia.* Reading, UK: Ithaca Press.

Zeitzen, M. K. (2008). *Polygamy. A cross cultural analysis.* Oxford, UK: Berg Publishers.

Teenage Marriage among Hmong American Women

Pa Der Vang
School of Social Work, St. Catherine University,
St. Paul, Minnesota, USA

Pa Her
Department of Social Science, New York City College of Technology,
Brooklyn, New York, USA

As Hmong transition to life in America, efforts are made by Hmong to maintain traditional cultural practices. This article explores the traditional practice of early marriage among Hmong women and their responses to this practice. As Hmong women acculturate to American ways, women may question the role of traditional practices in their identity and everyday lives. This study examines the family socialization and individual processes associated with teenage marriage among Hmong American women. Interviews with 12 Hmong American women who were married in their teens describe their experiences.

INTRODUCTION

Studies show that a significant number of Hmong American girls continue to enter into teenage marriages despite the negative consequences of early marriage on socioeconomic and mental health outcomes (Lee, Xiong, & Yuen, 2006; Vang & Bogenscutz, 2011a, 2011b). Women who marry in their teens, regardless of race, are more likely to report lower educational attainment, lower income, and increased mental health symptoms later in life (Burden & Klerman, 1984; Teti & Lamb, 1989; Moore et al., 1993; Upchurch, 1993; Astone & Upchurch, 1994; Sharlin, 1998; Vang & Bogenschutz, 2011a, 2011b). Among scholars, there is increased focus on the factors that underlie teenage marriages (Dahl, 2010). Because many Hmong women in the United States still tend to marry in their teens (Bays, 1994; Dunnigan, Onley, McNall, & Spring, 1996; Vang & Bogenschutz, 2011a, 2011b), there is a critical need to understand the processes that contribute to Hmong American women's entry into teenage marriage.

This study contributes to the literature by examining family socialization and individual processes related to teenage marriage among Hmong American women. Using narratives collected through semi-structured interviews, we examine family socialization experiences as well as familial values and beliefs that are transmitted from generation-to-generation to gain greater understanding of Hmong American women's insights and perspectives pertaining to teenage marriage.

Portions of this manuscript were presented at the Hmong Diaspora Institute on October 22, 2011, Madison, WI.

HMONG AMERICANS

Although there are debates as to where Hmong originated, research generally confirms that Hmong can be traced back as far as 2679 BC in China (Koltyk, 1998). The Hmong lived in the mountain areas in South China (Hamilton-Merritt, 1993). Their eventual displacement from China took place amid war and competition over economic resources in the 1800s. During this time of war and economic upheaval, a sizeable number of Hmong migrated to Southeast Asia while some stayed behind. The Hmong in Southeast Asia made their homes in countries such as Laos, Vietnam, Thailand, Burma, and Cambodia, and significant numbers continue to reside in these countries.

The Hmong in the United States are primarily from Laos, with small numbers from other countries as a result of secondary migration. The Hmong in Laos were recruited by U.S. CIA officials as soldiers in the Secret War, an effort to stop arms transport within Laos during the Vietnam War. Because of their role in the Secret War,[1] the Hmong in Laos were forced to flee their villages in fear of persecution and retaliation from communist regimes in Laos. The Hmong sought shelter in Thai refugee camps until they were later resettled to various countries such as Australia, Germany, France, Canada, and the United States (Center for Cross-Cultural Health, 2000). Since 1975, the Hmong population in the United States has quadrupled, making it one of the fastest-growing Southeast Asian ethnic groups. Currently, nearly 227,000 Hmong live in the United States, with the largest populations in California, Minnesota, and Wisconsin (American Community Survey [ACS], 2009).

Hmong have historically been identified as highland dwellers who preferred an agrarian lifestyle; planting their own food and raising livestock for a living. This agrarian lifestyle led to the formation and necessity of large families; more children meant more help on the farm. The developmental period of adolescence that is present in the United States and other industrialized countries did not exist for Hmong in Laos. Hmong children were typically given adult responsibilities as they moved from childhood to adolescence. This developmental period of adolescence for the Hmong is changing in the United States as a result of acculturation to an American lifestyle where adolescence is considered a pivotal stage in human development (Larson, Wilson, & Rickman, 2009).

Hmong Beliefs and Customs on Marriage

Teenage marriage has been an accepted practice among the Hmong for centuries (Downing, 1984; Hutchison & McNall, 1994; Lee, 1997; McNall, Dunnigan, & Mortimer, 1994; Ngo, 2002; Swartz, Lee, & Mortimer, 2003; Lee et al., 2006). For Hmong, marriage is a defining practice that forms social bonds and interdependence between two clans.[2] Because the Hmong place high value on the virtuousness of a bride, a younger bride was often preferred for there was a higher likelihood that she would be a virgin. Having a virtuous reputation also increased the likelihood that daughters would marry into a family with a good reputation, thus bonding her family of origin to a clan with a good reputation (a good reputation is one that denotes good genetic markers, wealth, or cleanliness and industriousness).

Hence, daughters were socialized early on for the next phase of life to be a wife and a daughter-in-law (Pho & Mulvey, 2003). Women who were not married by their late teens were considered "old maids" or unworthy of marriage (Thao, 1986; Donnelly, 1994; Symonds, 2004). Since the union of two clans reinforces an important virtue of interconnectedness and collectivism within Hmong society, teenage marriage remains intact in the United States despite the hindering consequences of this practice on the lives of Hmong American women (Lee et al., 2006; Vang & Bogenschutz, 2011a, 2011b).

In their countries of origin, marriage is a springboard into adulthood that occurred early in an agrarian society since the demand for labor left little time for adolescence (Symonds, 2004). Children in agrarian societies assumed early adult roles in order to contribute to the survival of the family. For daughters, this meant marriage soon after menses (Symonds, 2004). Brides contributed domestic labor to their husband's families while at the same time, as wives, women began bearing children soon after marriage, adding to the pool of labor supply available to her new family (Symonds, 2004). For parents of the bride, benefits came from marrying their daughter off early. Parents received a bride price paid by the groom's family as compensation for the labor that would be lost to the family if she were to marry. The bride price also symbolized respect for the parents' rearing of the daughter, her youth, and her virtuous status. In addition, teenage marriages were encouraged in order to prevent premarital pregnancies among teens: a time when the risk for premarital sex is typically high.

Scholars have argued in the United States that these traditional reasons for teenage marriage (i.e., marrying early to avoid spinsterhood and to maintain a virtuous reputation) are somewhat antiquated (Moua, 2003). However, most agree that teenage marriage in the United States continues among the Hmong, and the practice is carried out in much the same way as centuries before because it is ingrained in Hmong society. Though less is known about the precursors or causes that promote teenage marriage, we argue there may be different incentives or motivators that encourage teenage marriage in the United States. For example, the traditional practice of having the young couple reside with the husband's family may have reinforced the value of maintaining a strong family unit; however, when teenage couples are provided food and shelter by family, teenagers do not face the fear that they must somehow fend for themselves in a labor-based wage-dependent economy. Having no housing costs may in effect neutralize the economic responsibilities of marriage because the couple can live together free of any housing costs to them. Additionally, when the couple gives birth to their first child; parent, grandparents and siblings all living within the same household may be available to help raise the child, thus freeing up the young couple's time. The young couple also avoids any child care costs in this type of living situation. Last, since most Hmong families arrive in the United States with little to no education, the bride price may act as a financial incentive for parents who could gain upwards of $5,000 per daughter. The paucity of research in this area suggests it is important to investigate other potential reasons that may account for teenage marriage in the United States.

Prevalence

Compared to non-Hmong groups in the United States, Hmong American women tend to marry between 11 years and 23 years of age (Bays, 1994; Dunnigan et al., 1996). However, the actual rate of teenage marriage among Hmong Americans is unclear due to the lack of studies in this area. Among the small study samples with Hmong American girls and women, reports of disparate teenage marriage rates ranged from 30% to 80% (Downing, 1984; Meschke, 2003; Swartz et al., 2003). For instance, McNall and colleagues (1994) found that almost 50% of Hmong high school students in a Midwestern state were married. Ten years later, the rate of teenage marriage remained unchanged; in a 2003 report distributed by the Lao Family of Minnesota, a non-profit organization serving Hmong, found that 50% of the 187 Hmong high school girls in their study were married (Meschke, 2003). Similarly, Swartz and colleagues (2003) found that 70% of students were married as teens in their study of educational achievement among Hmong girls. More recently, Vang and Bogenschutz (2011a, 2011b), using a sample size of 186 Hmong women over the age of 18, reported that 31.7% of the women in their study were married at age 17 or younger. These studies suggest that Hmong teenage marriages continue in the United States, and more research needs to be conducted to understand this phenomenon.

CONCEPTUAL FRAMEWORK

Our conceptual framework that may help explain Hmong American women's paths into teenage marriage stems from social learning theories (Bandura, 1977; Mischel, 1973; Sears, 1975) and examines the role of culture that is transmitted through the family. Culture of origin is an influential factor that shapes one's values and beliefs. Perhaps the most direct way to learn about cultural values and practices is through family socialization processes (Cole & Tan, 2007), as marriage is a part of early human socialization. Theories of social learning emphasize the importance of observing and modeling the behaviors, attitudes, and emotional reactions of others. That is, from a social learning perspective, marriage during the teenage years and raising children in multigenerational households is normative in some communities because they have observed other models (e.g., parents, sisters, cousins, close friends) engage in teenage marriages and witnessed the consequences thereof. The consequences of teenage marriage such as early pregnancy, dropping out of high school, and seeking social welfare benefits became normative as they witness several models follow this sequence. Another line of argument similar among other ethnic minorities is that with little encouragement or few role models to identify with, Hmong women may feel that education and labor force opportunities are out of reach (Stevens-Simon & Lowy, 1995) and, therefore, choose to adopt roles that are more readily accessible such as early marriage within a traditional cultural context.

Other potential factors may contribute toward teenage marriage include not only culture and unique familial experiences but also one's individual insights and perspectives (i.e., reasoning or motivation). However, these individual processes are influenced by messages received from within the family system. How one understands their experiences reflects the teachings or socialization from within the family system, including the extended family. Therefore, we examine the messages learned from within the family and extended family as it relates to Hmong women's own insights and perspectives.

We acknowledge that the entire environment includes not only the microsystem, but also mezzo- and macro-environmental factors. However, we focus on microsystem experiences of the family as the family experiences have one of the most direct influences on children's outcomes. We do, however, discuss how these micro-level experiences may interact with the individual's experiences with the mezzo- and macro-systems and the participants' perceptions of these experiences. Hmong girls who choose teenage marriage face many barriers to success in their American context (Lee et al., 2006; Vang & Bogenschutz, 2011a), an experience that is foreign to their mothers or grandmothers who lived a mono-cultural existence until their entry into the United States. In their home countries, Hmong women who married young face the same issues as Hmong teenage brides in the United States. Therefore, the experiences of Hmong girls who marry early in the United States, although normed within their own familial setting, are out of the norm when compared to social norms set by mainstream mezzo- and macro-systems. Focusing on the interaction between micro- and macro-systems, the goal of the present study was to examine socialization processes, including direct observations, family normaliziation, and verbal socialization of teenage marriage as it relates to Hmong women's insights and perspectives.

METHODS

This study was approved by the IRB of California State University-San Bernardino. Because of the paucity of research in this area, the present study served as an exploratory pilot study to inform future intervention and/or research studies. These in-depth qualitative narratives with 12 Hmong American women who were married under the age of 18 may enhance our understanding of the kinds of changes in family practices that would be particularly maladaptive or adaptive within a specific cultural context. The 12 participants were recruited through several means. First, a recruitment notice was posted on a Hmong women's online forum used by many members of the Hmong community. Due to increased access to technology, many Hmong communicate via the Internet. Via this online forum, participants were recruited through word of mouth by other participants that resulted in snowball sampling. Data were collected via semi-structured interviews. The researcher met each woman in her home. Each interview lasted anywhere between 1.5 hours and 2 hours.

The research questions for this study encourage participants to discuss ways in which they were socialized by family and peers as well as their individual insights and perspectives related to their early marriages. Using an interview guide, the research asked participants questions about their beliefs and values regarding marriage learned in childhood, the family and peer values they were exposed to about womanhood, the circumstances surrounding the participants' marriage, their family and community response to their early marriage, and their own insights pertaining to their marital situation. All interviews were recorded and transcribed by the researcher. Interviews were coded according to major themes that surfaced from the data (Glaser & Strauss, 1967).

RESULTS AND DISCUSSION

The 12 participants varied between ages 22 and 39. Five of the women were born in either Laos or Thailand, while seven were born in the United States. Participants were married between the ages of 14 and 17. Participants resided in various states representative of Hmong communities in the United States, including six from Minnesota, three from California, and one from Wisconsin, one from North Carolina, and one from Georgia. The areas with the highest population of Hmong are the Twin Cities metro of Minnesota, Central Valley areas of California, and the Fox Valley areas of Wisconsin.

The two broad themes reflecting social learning theories were found in the data: (1) family socialization processes and (2) individual insight and perspectives. Each theme is further delineated by more specific themes and will be discussed in further detail (Table 1). The themes are intended to highlight the manner in which Hmong American women are socialized toward teenage marriage through family socialization processes and their own individual insights and perspectives for engaging in teenage marriage. These themes inform practitioners of the experiences of Hmong American women when engaging teenage marriage and are intended to provide a foundation for discussing marriage with Hmong girls and women.

The first theme—family socialization processes—refers to the subtle messages within families that shape the norms and values surrounding overt and covert behaviors of each family member. These messages become internalized. Many individuals live out these messages in everyday life unquestioningly. However, some individuals possess the self-awareness and insight to ques-

TABLE 1
Family Socialization and Individual Insight and Perspectives

Major Themes	Sub-Themes
Family Socialization Processes	a. Observational learning of teenage marriages: Direct Observation of Teenage Marriage Involving Family Members
	b. Family Discourse
	c. Primary Socialization
Individual Insight and Perspectives	
1. Internalization of Cultural Practices	a. High acceptance
	b. Low acceptance
2. Escape-avoidance	a. Affirmation
	b. Disappointment

tion the norms and values passed down by family. The second theme—individual insights and perspectives—refers to the uniqueness of each individual and her ability to be critical of her own situations. Individual insights make it possible for individuals to analyze messages learned from their family and challenge the norms and values that may not fit with their own individual perspectives.

FAMILY SOCIALIZATION PROCESSES

The women interviewed described several factors contributing to their decision to marry as teenagers. In common with all participants were explicit and implicit messages from their families and extended relatives and peers normalizing teenage marriage. All messages about teenage marriage endorsed the plausibility of teenage marriage for young daughters, thus socializing Hmong daughters to accept teenage marriage as a viable option in their own lives. These messages were categorized under "family socialization processes" and included both implicit and explicit messages. These socialization processes were carried out through three primary processes: (1) direct observation of teenage marriages involving their own family members (these being implicit messages), (2) a family discourse that normalized teenage marriage (explicit messages), and (3) verbal socialization toward teenage marriage (explicit messages) such as explicit messages from parents and relatives regarding certain behaviors that would make a daughter more appealing for marriage. Each subtheme is discussed separately in the following section.

Direct Observation of Teenage Marriage Involving Family Members

Nine participants (75%) stated that in their early childhood and early adolescence, they attended the marriage ceremonies of their older female cousins or sisters who were in their middle- to late-adolescent ages at the time. Observing their sister or a close other adolescent participate in teenage marriage made the practice seem acceptable or normal for most of the participants.

> I don't remember anyone ever saying anything about my cousin's young age. It was just not an issue. It was normal to everyone and to me at the time ...

> When I was younger most of my cousins got married early. I just thought that's what girls were supposed to do when you reach that age since everyone else was doing it.

> I remember one time one of my cousins got married to a girl from another town. The girl was just a little older than me.... When they got married, I don't remember anyone ever saying anything about her age but she was just a teenager too. I guess it was just so normal that no one ever thought it was different.

The participants' observation of family members' marriages is reflected in these two statements. Their narratives reflect their perception, at the time, that marriage in adolescence seemed normal; almost a rite of passage for girls this age. Here, there are no explicit messages about teenage marriage, but their observation and participation in the ceremony suggest that their immediate environment supports the practice. These statements also suggest a lack of perceived negative consequences or lack of inhibition toward teenage marriage and the notion that teenage marriage is acceptable. In addition, the participants rely on their observations of others' lived experiences to guide their decision. At the same time, the narratives indicate that participants felt that it was their duty to become married at a particular age. As conformity to peers peaks during early adolescence (Eccles, 1999), this type of observational learning from family members may significantly impact one's decision to marry during her teenage years based on social acceptance rather than deliberate decision.

Family Culture Normalizing Teenage Marriage

A majority of the women (75%) interviewed identified messages conveyed to them by their immediate and extended family about teenage marriage as a common and accepted occurrence, a daughter's role in the family and community, and the notion that marriage during adolescence is a normal and encouraged rite of passage for teens. The acceptability of teenage marriage was conveyed verbally through family stories and in the everyday language used by the family. The reality of teenage marriage was a part of the family discourse and cultural norm, thus exposing participants to the notion of marriage at an early age. The statements made by the participants reflected aspects of family life that normalized teenage marriage. These include

> Throughout my childhood, I remember my mom, aunts, and grandmother sitting around talking about my female cousins who were married. Sometimes my aunts would also talk about their daughters-in-law. I never really thought about it, but now that we're talking about it, even at my young age, I was aware that these girls were still teenagers.

> My brother got married when I was younger. They lived with us for about three years.... My sister-in-law was just about 16 or so I think and she went to high school. My brother used to drive us all to school.

The statements above demonstrate how Hmong families across generations engage in open discussions about their daughters and/or granddaughters who married as teenagers. When children hear and participate in these discussions, they start to internalize that notion that teenage marriage is acceptable. In this sense, the cultural norms of the family are expressed through verbal storytelling. These stories transmit cultural beliefs and values to children who may be more eager to mimic adult ways. The women do not question the "normalcy" of teenage marriage in their own upbringing. Their experiences with teenage marriage within their immediate families and extended family system may support a developing belief that teenage marriage is a life-event that could actually occur during their own teenage years.

At other times, marriage appears to be the only alternative in cases of unplanned pregnancies for a teen-aged Hmong woman. Traditionally, Hmong families would not allow teenager daughters to become a single parent due to the shame and loss of face associated with this practice. In addition, termination of the pregnancy is rarely discussed because it was not an option available in an agrarian society. However, single teen mothers and abortions are becoming more common as the Hmong acculturate to Western society. Traditionally, marriage is especially likely if the father is also Hmong as Hmong families tend to hold the father of the child responsible by forcing marriage (Fontes, 2005). Marriage in this way saves the family's reputation and resolves the shame associated with having an unmarried pregnant daughter. The benefits of saving the family's and her own reputation in this collectivistic society may trump the needs and individual wishes of their daughter. Thus, in cases of teenage marriage due to unplanned pregnancy, observers of this practice learn that marriage is the more socially acceptable option because it serves to protect the family's reputation:

> One of my cousins got pregnant when she was in high school and she was forced to marry. She was 16 ... I don't think there was another choice for her ... um ... at least I don't remember because what I remember is that she got pregnant and she had to get married.

Finally, all participants ($N = 12$) reported that their own mothers were married as teenagers. Family stories that include notions of teenage marriage serve as a mechanism to normalize the idea of teenage marriage within the family culture. For example, one interviewee stated,

> Well, I just remember my mom telling us stories of how she got married to my dad. She was really young too. Back then they didn't know their birthdays but she said she was still just a young girl.

Here we see family stories that contribute to the formation of culture as they imagine and reproduce ethnic identity through their mother's own stories as a young bride (Langellier, 2002). Because parents, especially mothers with their daughters, serve as important role models for learning appropriate behavior, the stories that mothers choose to discuss with their daughters may be one way teenage Hmong American women become socialized into teenage marriages.

Verbal Socialization of Girls toward Teenage Marriage

Coupled with indirect forms of socialization, direct socialization of marriage through cultural messages of what it means to be a "good wife" and "nyab" (*daughter in law, pronounced "nya"*) from primary agents of socialization (i.e., parents, and close relatives) plays an important role in shaping the values and beliefs of marriage. Participants reported that their parents and relatives would consistently convey messages that a Hmong girl must learn how to be a good wife or face spinsterhood. These cultural messages of what it means to be a "good wife" reinforces the patriarchal organization of the Hmong family system:

> When I was younger, I remember my parents always telling me that I had to learn how to be a good wife and they used to say things like "if you don't get married when you're still young, no one will want to marry you when you're old."

> I learned how to cook at a very young age. I think I was in fifth grade when I cooked my very first meal for the family. I remember how happy my dad was that I was able to do this. My parents would say things to me about how to be a good nyab. They would say things like, "If you burn the rice they won't like you."

> One time I was throwing a fit and my dad said, "You're going to be a nyab and you're acting like that? No one is going to want you to be their nyab. They'll probably send you back to us."[3]

Messages that place emphasis on learning domestication skills such as cooking and marrying at an early age are reflected in these statements. Particularly, the statement by one Hmong woman's parents "no one will want to marry you when you're old" suggests that one should marry early or face a life of spinsterhood. The "natural" unfolding of Hmong maturity is to be married with children, and this encouragement may subsequently lead to earlier Hmong marriages and pressures for childbirth before they reach their eighteenth birthday (Lo, 2002). Here, learning domestication skills is conveyed as adding value to your role as a daughter, wife, and mother, in turn; these skills will gain you social approval from others, especially your family, and your future in-laws.

Extrinsic rewards such as gaining approval or praises or avoiding "*being sent back*" to her family may motivate girls to engage and stay in teenage marriage. The message suggests that she may bring shame to her family and the clan because she did not act accordingly. It is not just encouragement or passing down these cultural messages but also parents' reinforcement of these "good" wife behaviors: "I remember how happy my dad was that I was able to do this . . . cook." Rather than simply passing down cultural message of what is "good" or "bad," here the parents also give positive praise for acting accordingly. Because this praise and advice stem from parents or important others, young girls may likely begin to seek ways to continue to earn this praise and social approval. Together, these multiple socialization experiences provide them with an awareness of socially ascribed roles.

INDIVIDUAL INSIGHT AND PERSPECTIVE

According to theoretical approaches, parents' beliefs and goals guide parents' socialization behaviors and, ultimately, contribute to their children's outcomes (Dix, 1991). Over time, repeated exposure to parents' socialization strategies is likely to influence children's own values and belief system. We discuss two broad individual cognitive processes reflected in the insights and perspectives shared by the participants: (1) internalization of cultural practice, including high acceptance (16.6%; $n = 2$) and low acceptance (75%; $n = 9$) and (2) escape-avoidance, including affirmation and disappointment (8.3%; $n = 1$).

Internalization of Cultural Practice

Internalization refers to the process of acceptance of a set of norms established by people or groups that are influential to the individual (Greenberg & Cheselka, 1995). Through direct observations of teenage marriage, the person first becomes aware of the set of values and norms. Awareness is followed by an understanding of the set of values or norms. This awareness may be a result of the socialization processes described earlier. As experiences accumulate and family members reinforce teenage marriage, the person moves toward adoption of these cultural values. Thus, the final stage is acceptance of the values or norms into one's own viewpoint. Individuals are not fully aware of the process of internalization.

All participants reported some level of internalization of teenage marriage as a concept within their own worldviews, meaning the manner in which they viewed the world included the concept of teenage marriage as a reality. The women in the study seemed to be aware of their internalization of teenage marriage on differing levels, and most were able to reflect on the impact of teenage marriage on their life. However, participants varied in their level of acceptance of teenage marriage. Some individuals exhibited high acceptance (16.6%; $n = 2$) while others reported low acceptance (75%; $n = 9$) of the practice of teenage marriage.

Individuals with high acceptance (16.6%; $n = 2$) of teenage marriage tended to speak of teenage marriage as an ordinary fact of life. These individuals reported satisfaction in their marriage, and a sense of pride about fulfilling the societal expectations of a Hmong woman. In fact, as a researcher, it felt intrusive at times to be asking questions about teenage marriage of women who had low insight about their internalization. For women who had accepted teenage marriage as a normal facet of their culture, teenage marriage appeared to be a way of life, reporting contentment and satisfaction with having been married as a teen. Acceptance was demonstrated by the absence of objection to having marriage as a teenager. Instead, participants spoke about their experiences using matter-of-fact language. It was not this researcher's position to question the participants' perceptions of their life situations since that is judgmental and leading.

A majority of participants (75%; $n = 9$) appeared to be unclear about their feelings about teenage marriage. Their interviews reflected a sense of ambivalence as well as low acceptance of teenage marriage. These individuals appeared to face an internal struggle regarding their participation and own feelings about teenage marriage as a practice. In addition, these participants reported a sense of loss in regard to the loss of their teenage years in lieu of early adulthood and the loss of personal choice in decisions about their life path and marriage. There appeared a sense of powerlessness in the stories shared by these women.

> Well I think marrying as a teenager really took away a lot. I mean I didn't get the chance to know myself, develop an identity, and now that my kids are grown, I'm getting that chance I think, but it's not the same. That's what marrying early does, girls don't get a chance to be a young adult because you start having kids and all the other responsibilities. . . .

> If I could do things differently, I don't think I would have married so young. I don't want my girls to make the same mistake. I want them to experience life while they are young before they get married.

The above emphasizes the importance of adolescence as a time for teenagers to develop a sense of identity that will serve as a basis for their adult lives according to Western worldview (Erikson,

1968). In the United States, teenagers who adopt adult roles prematurely and assume adult responsibilities before identity issues are resolved may, as adults, grieve their lost adolescence. Here, adopting the role of wife and mother "took away a lot," where she does not feel that the loss can be replaced. As a result of this loss of identity, these women may display ambivalence towards their decision to marry.

> Back then you didn't know any better. You just thought since everyone else is getting married that you should get married. It's kind of sad how girls get into that situation and then they realize later what they did. I feel like I never really got to learn about myself.

> You know, you just marry because some man wants to marry you and you don't realize what you're doing until it's too late. Life has been good but it could have been different.

As Hmong women contemplate the impact of these lost adolescent years, conflict in marriages may result, leading to higher rates of divorce among Hmong teenage brides (Vang & Bogenschutz, 2013).

In these narratives, the concept of identity comes into play repeatedly, but decision-making abilities also matter. Shown here, a key point for engaging in teenage marriage is social approval because "some man wants to marry you" and "everyone else was getting married" are reasons for getting married in your teens. However, at this time, adolescents have lower abstract reasoning abilities to think about the future, and this lack of reasoning may lead them to choose more immediately rewarding decisions than those that require time and education (Baron & Brown, 1991). Teens may also need more experimentation with different identities before committing to adult roles (Erickson, 1968) to develop a concrete sense of identity.

In addition, some women with low acceptance demonstrated a desire to make the best out of their situation with statements such as

> Sometimes if you cause trouble[4] you have to stick it out and take responsibility for what you've gotten yourself into.

> Well, I guess you just take what life gives you and you do your best. Overall, I think it's been good, but there are days when you wonder what if. . . .

One interpretation from above is that these women are resilient even when they express a desire for a different life situation and despite the acknowledgement of the possible losses (e.g., education, identity, experiences). Rather than focusing on their sense of loss, their narratives reflect an effort to change their perspectives of the situation by endorsing that they did what they could to improve their lives and continue to make the best of their marriages. They understood the situation in a positive meaning in light of the losses they reported. These statements suggest that strong ties to their culture of origin mitigated the effects of losses they experienced in adolescence. The rewards provided by the culture of origin for being a good wife and daughter compensated for the losses that might have been perceived as a Westernized adolescent. However, their statements also allude to another potential explanation we turn to next.

That is, these young girls may have internalized feelings of inferiority due to their ascribed roles and "daughter, wife, mother, *nyab*" and may not learn to develop their active agency or their own independent voice (Belenky, Clinchy, Goldberger, & Tarule, 1986). By speaking up, they are only "causing trouble" for themselves. It is the intersections of these various marginalized positions, along with their internalized inferiority, that have socialized them to be passive rather than seeking a change. These women may accept the messages and try to live up to the standards of the motherhood mandate and social scripts regarding collectivism and family honor passed on by the "knowledgeable."

Escape-Avoidance

The last sub-theme within the theme individual insight and perspective was escape-avoidance. This type of individual coping strategy is characterized by the effort to escape from having to deal with a stressor like a negative home environment (Folkman, 1984). Three women shared that marrying in the teenage years was a way to escape or avoid their current home environment in search for a better one. These women described demanding and unhappy home environments in childhood that ultimately led to their decisions to marry in their teens. They discussed their home environments as those in which they were assigned multiple household responsibilities and where they were obligated to assume adult roles in the home. Household responsibilities included providing care for younger siblings, cleaning, and assuming sole responsibility for preparing meals for the family on a daily basis. Traditionally, Hmong families assign the duties of cooking and cleaning to the females in the home. Responsibilities for cooking rested heavily on mother and oldest daughter. Cooking responsibilities can be substantial as Hmong families typically have five to six children and grandparents living in one household.

> It was a way out for me. My dad very abusive ... not only that, I had to come home from school every day and watch my nieces and nephews, cook, and my parents never let me do anything. I met my husband at school when I was thirteen and he would visit me at home for two years. He felt so bad for me ... when he was about to move away he asked me to marry him. I was only fifteen.

These substantial responsibilities in the home and parents' strict control over their daughters' whereabouts prevented daughters from socializing with peers and blocked their ability to partic-ipate in autonomy-seeking activities in adolescence. Autonomy-seeking behaviors include those such as taking a part-time job, extracurricular activities such as sports and arts, and volunteering among others that expose adolescents to a gradual entrance into adulthood in the United States. Marriage was seen as an entry into adulthood and freedom from strict control of parents.

Within the escape-avoidance theme, participants' expectation for finding a better situation through marriage were either *affirmed* or they were *disappointed*, and they found themselves in situations that were either worse or no better than life with their own parents. Participants whose desire to escape was affirmed reported a newfound sense of independence soon after the marriage. These participants reported marrying into families who were supportive and where strong emotional bonds were forged with the husband's siblings and other daughters-in-law who also resided in the house. These women reported having positive relationships with their spouses. In addition, these women reported fulfilled autonomy and independence in the form of moving out of the in-laws' home with their spouses early on and feeling successful in accomplishing milestones in their lives with their spouses including having children, completing their educational goals, and eventually becoming a home owner.

> I got along with my sister-in-laws. And his mom was pretty nice to me. He took me to school every day and they didn't have a problem that I had to study at night because my sister-in-law was in school too. I don't think it was a big deal for me.

> We only lived with them for two years and we were able to move out on our own. Umm, and ... we got an apartment when he got a full time job. His parents never had a problem with it, I don't think. They treated me like a daughter and they kept to themselves most of the time.

Women who reported disappointment in fulfilling their hopes of escaping the negative environ-ments within their families of origin reported marrying into families who were equally as verbally and emotionally abusive as their own families (no physical abuse by the in-laws was reported). These women found themselves having to assume similar parentified responsibilities, if not more, as they had when living with their birth parents. In traditional Hmong families, daughters-in-law are assigned substantial domestic duties upon marrying. These include cooking, cleaning, caring for younger children in the home, caring for aged in-laws, and bearing several children of their own. In addition, these women reported unsupportive or unsatisfying relationships with their spouses. The husbands of these women often endorsed cultural views and beliefs that supported the subordination of women.

> At first I had to do a lot. I watched my husband's younger brothers and sisters. I did a lot of things like, um, come home from school and cook dinner for everyone. It wasn't easy. I didn't have a lot of time for homework.

> We got pregnant right away. Back then I didn't know any better. I didn't think about those kinds of things. You just get pregnant and do what they ask you to do ... um ... I just took over doing things like a lot of daughters-in-laws do, you know, do all the cooking and cleaning and basically, they just got a new helping hand you know.

> He was not very supportive. He always sided with his mom whenever we had an argument. It was hard ... he is very typical in that he wanted me to be the submissive wife and I couldn't do that because I was in school and I was very involved in things at school.

Unfortunately, for these women, their hope of finding new independence with their spouse was met with disappointment as they found themselves shouldering even heavier familial duties as a daughter-in-law. With little to no support, these women reported disappointment and ambivalence in their decision to marry early as teens.

IMPLICATIONS OF STUDY

The narratives from these qualitative interviews highlight beliefs and socialization phenomena pertaining to the practice of teenage marriage. Contrary to how daughters in mainstream American society are socialized toward marriage in adulthood, many Hmong American daughters are socialized in their immediate family to marry in their teens. Socialization practices leading to the internalization of beliefs surrounding traditional marriage practices among Hmong American women serve as major contributing factors for the high rates of teenage marriage in the Hmong community within the United States Specifically, our study shows that family socialization strategies can reinforce cultural and family values about teenage marriage, thereby influencing their daughters' perceptions endorsing teenage marriage and an internalized belief that normalizes the practice of teenage marriage. There appeared to be a variety of reasons for teenage marriage, including more traditional and individual motivators.

It is important to avoid judgment or negative labeling of family socialization practices pertaining to teenage marriage. In addition, questioning client's acceptance of teenage marriage may create confusion for the client. Instead, practitioners must help Hmong American women gain insight into the role of teenage marriage as a cultural practice within their lives in the context of mainstream American society. Girls must develop an awareness of the influence of the culturally specific construction of teenage marriage on their own decision-making process. In addition, girls must develop an awareness of cultural differences pertaining to institutions of marriage.

Practice Interventions

Social workers who work with Hmong women and girls must seek education about traditional marriages practices within the Hmong community. Social workers must work with cultural consultants who can provide valuable information and act as liaisons with Hmong families. Social workers must be considerate of the self-determination of Hmong girls while at the same time being respectful of cultural traditions of Hmong. The primary goal is to work toward the best interest of the client. It is the social worker's responsibility to inform the young girl of the consequences of her decisions whether she chooses to marry early or not, while encouraging the girl to make the final decision. It is important that the social worker ensure that the girl has received the information she needs such as consequences of actions and alternative choices before she makes a decision; the decision must be one that is informed. Thus, it is important that social workers obtain education about traditional Hmong marriage in order to work effectively with Hmong girls faced with this decision. Social workers must suspend their judgment and opinion about teenage marriage and try not to influence the situation according to how they feel about teenage marriage. Finally, social workers must be able to talk about teenage marriage with Hmong girls without blame or shame of the young girls; in addition, the social worker must not use the intervention with the girl as a means to resolving his or her own countertransference surrounding teenage marriage. In this next section, we make a suggestion for direct practice intervention with Hmong girls.

Narrative therapy, developed by social workers Michael White and David Epston, allows individuals to examine social constructs that have shaped their lives by separating the person from these social and mental processes (White, 2004). The narrative approach does not negate or label the stories of Hmong American women; rather, the narrative approach explores the family and cultural stories that have shaped their identity. A narrative approach assumes that the provider first possess a complex understanding of teenage marriage within Hmong culture, that acknowledges and validates the lived experiences of their clients.[5]

The narrative approach also utilizes the strategy of *externalization*. In its original form, externalization approaches a "problem" existent in the client's life such as alcoholism or depression and externalizes it by using language that removes the problem from the person's identity. For example, rather than speaking of alcoholism as "your alcoholism," the therapist would state "let's talk about alcoholism." An externalization technique is recommended that similarly separates the concept of teenage marriage from the identity of a Hmong woman will allow the client to examine the concept of teenage marriage objectively. This practice challenges Western therapists to be grounded and to challenge their own comfort level. Often times, Western therapists believe that to be culturally sensitive is to talk about culturally specific concepts using non-judgmental language; to act as if teenage marriage were a normal everyday part of life in order to sound non-judgmental. The researchers suggest that in order to use narrative therapy, the practitioner must name the issue head on. That is, the practitioner must be comfortable enough to discuss teenage marriage, including the pros and cons of teenage marriage in an objective manner. Thus, the therapist must be able to say to the client, "Let's talk about teenage marriage" without feeling as though they are being disrespectful to their client.

The narrative approach encourages therapists to name the issue at hand, openly and directly. The first author's own counseling experience with Hmong women who were faced with the decision to marry in their teens has used this approach by openly talking about the issue in a genuine, curious, and empathetic manner. The narratives shown in the current study suggest that these women may not be consciously aware about the cultural conflict of teenage marriage. Although several participants briefly noted that teenage marriage directly conflicted with the norms surrounding adolescence in American culture, none elaborated on it.

Narrative therapy techniques may encourage Hmong women to discuss teenage marriage because it removes the notion of teenage marriage and the problems assigned to it by Western culture from their identity, giving women the permission to discuss marriage without feeling as though they are overexposed to an outsider and possibly making their own personal identities vulnerable to judgment. It is recommended that the therapist identify contrasting and comparable aspects of both the host American culture and Hmong culture to reveal the plethora of life choices available to the client. Comparing and contrasting these two cultures should not be made in the tone that feels as though the therapist is trying to sway the client toward Western culture or somehow contrasting to see which decision is better. The point of talking about these two differing cultures is to help the client envision two possible life stories: a way to encourage her to craft a life story for herself. Social workers can also use the narrative approach to assist clients in co-constructing emergent life stories.

Focusing on the clients' personal experiences and how these experiences have shaped the lives and thought patterns of the clients will assist the social worker in developing a thorough intervention plan that is inclusive of the client's culture of origin. The co-construction of life stories must include not only the clients' lived experiences within their own culture but within dominant culture as well; assisting clients in creating a new life story that combines the realities of both cultures. In addition, the social worker must take into account client self determination while at the same time providing guidance in sorting out the many facets of Hmong American women's lived experiences in the United States, lives that embrace two cultures.

Policy Interventions

Hmong marriage takes place in a traditional cultural ceremony. The ceremony does not occur within legal sanction from any legal or court system in the United States; therefore, a Hmong girl can be married without legal systems' being aware of the underage marriage. Hmong marriages are conducted by a mej koob (pronounced may-kong) who officiates the marriage and facilitates the negotiations between the two families. The mej koob is a member of the clan. The traditional marriage is considered an official marriage by members of the Hmong community although it has not been officiated by the American court. Once the couple turns 18, they may then decide to officiate their marriage in a court of law. Many times, couples never officiate their marriage, and they run into problems related to property rights when there is a divorce or death. Traditional marriage ceremonies not only exist in Hmong culture but are also a part of many other cultures. In the United States, European-style marriages have been institutionalized within our social and legal structure; however, our society has failed to legally recognize the traditional marriage practice of other cultures. By providing legal recognition to traditional Hmong marriages, our society may be able to prevent teenage marriages among the Hmong. By providing legal sanction to traditional marriage practices, the state can then provide legal sanctions around the legal age of marriage within traditional marriage practices. In the state of Minnesota, such as the Hmong Marriage Bill (HF 3674; SF 2403) was introduced in the Minnesota Legislature in 2006 to solemnize Hmong marriages. The bill would require the mej koob to file papers with the American court system to officiate the marriage. This bill would have expanded the law making it a form of neglect to allow minors to marry by requiring that the mej koob report underage marriage to Child Protection authorities (MN State Legislature, 2006). The Hmong marriage bill drew heated debate in the Hmong community. Some members of the community were wary of giving government control of traditional Hmong marriages, while some members of the community believed that legal recognition of traditional Hmong marriages would legitimize a very important traditional practice within Hmong culture. The bill was tabled for further study in 2006 with hopes that it would be revisited in 2007. However, the bill was not moved forward in 2007.

Because our legal systems have less awareness of traditional marriage among many underage Hmong girls, these situations rarely come to the attention of child protection systems. Although many child protection agencies have encountered underage marriage among Hmong girls, more proactive measures must be put in place to address the situation. Hmong girls who marry early are forced to grow up quickly. These girls do not have the opportunity to experience adolescent identity development, which may result in poor sense of self and poor mental health outcomes in the future (Vang & Bogenschutz, 2011). Many times, teenage girls are married to much older men, which would warrant intervention by child protection in states where statutory rape laws are applicable.

Research Interventions

There are no large-scale studies on the prevalence of teenage marriage among the Hmong in the United States or worldwide. A study of this nature is necessary in order to give researchers and policy makers the information needed to plan interventions for women facing this situation. Current studies rely on small samples.

Further research is also needed to understand the impact of teenage marriage on multiple systems in the lives of these young Hmong women while also being considerate of the loss of traditional practices for Hmong. As the traditional practice of teenage marriage becomes increasingly challenged by American systems, the Hmong community must grapple with the loss of a century-old tradition. This concept of culture loss must be further explored for its impact on members of the Hmong community and Hmong girls. In regard to impacts on women's lives, as Hmong women delay marriage in pursuit of education and employment, they will find it more difficult to find a mate within the Hmong community who will accept them. In the Hmong community, young women who are more likely to be subservient to their husband are considered more appealing for marriage than an older more educated Hmong woman. Young to middle adult women with educations and careers are viewed as threats to the patriarchy, who may emasculate their husbands and fail to obey traditions.

Finally, more research is needed to understand the interventions utilized by Child Protection Systems and public schools in response to teenage marriage among Hmong girls. Little information can be found regarding how public systems are responding to these situations and what decisions are being made surrounding the ethical dilemma systems must face as they grapple with how to intervene to the best interest of the young girl. This type of research would provide valuable educational materials for practicing social workers and agencies who work with Hmong women and girls.

STRENGTHS, LIMITATIONS, AND CONCLUSION

Our study makes several contributions to the literature. First, we provide new information on Hmong Americans, a rapidly growing and understudied group in the United States. Next, we explored the experiences and beliefs of an immigrant group facing cultural change as they transition to life in a host country. And third, we discuss cultural practices that may have held symbolic meaning in another place and time but are currently being challenged in a new society and the implications for social work.

We note three limitations to this study in particular. First, and perhaps most important, our small sample size suggests lack of generalizability. Within-group variation is essential to consider, especially one's acculturation level as it may relate to different beliefs about marriage (Lee et al., 2009). The participants of this study were raised in families led by first-generation refugee parents. Thus, the family backgrounds of participants may be more consistent with traditional Hmong culture. It is also important to acknowledge that first-generation Hmong parents also vary in their beliefs about teenage marriage, views on childrearing, and their level of ascription to dominant individualistic views. Future work incorporating larger samples will be critical for understanding mechanisms underlying teenage marriage. Second, self-selection may influence the findings of this study; women who chose to participate are more willing to openly discuss their perspective on teenage marriage, thus excluding the viewpoints of women who may have had completely different experiences. Future studies including diverse experiences will be important. Third, multiple pathways for teenage marriage manifested in participants in divergent ways, with some women indicating contentment or positive experiences whereas others experienced ambivalence or uncertainty about their decision to marry as a teenager. In the case of Hmong American women, living life within two cultures may contribute to conflicting experiences and views regarding teenage marriage. Overall, this study sheds light on the influence of culture and family on Hmong American women's decisions to marry in their teens. Socializations experiences communicate family and cultural values and beliefs that influence the lives of clients. We have examined potential precursors and mechanisms that may be associated with teenage marriage, including family socialization and individual processes. Strategies from narrative therapy such as externalization may aid social workers in discussing this sensitive yet important topic with Hmong girls.

NOTES

1. The Hmong were recruited as soldiers in the "Secret War," a U.S.-backed effort against communism in Laos.
2. Hmong families are members of 1 of only 18 clans and have one of the only 18 surnames (McInnis, Share all of the surnames 1991). All 18 clans are represented in the United States.
3. In Hmong marriage practices, the husband may send the new bride back to her parents' home, signifying the initiation of a divorce resulting in loss of face for the young woman and her parents.
4. The participant used the phrase "cause trouble" to refer to the act of taking on adult responsibilities at such a young age.
5. This recommendation is consistent with the NASW Code of Ethics (2008) statement of responsibility to clients in the area cultural competency and social diversity. The NASW Code of Ethics (2008) suggests that social workers develop an understanding of the client's culture and the function of culture in the client's life and their interaction with society.

REFERENCES

American Community Survey. (2009). *2005–2007 American Community Survey Hmong Population Data*. Retrieved from http://www.census.gov/acs/www/index.html

Astone, N. M.. & Upchurch, D. M. (1994). Forming a family, leaving school early, earning a G.E.D.: A racial and cohort comparison. *Journal of Marriage & Family*, *56*(3), 759–772.

Bandura, A. (1977) *Social learning theory*. Englewood Cliffs, NJ: Prentice Hall.

Baron, J., & Brown, R.V. (1991). Toward improved instruction in decision making to adolescents: A conceptual framework and pilot program. In J. Baron & R. V. Brown (Eds.), *Teaching decision making to adolescents* (pp. 95–122). Hillsdale, NJ: Lawrence Erlbaum Associates.

Bays, S. (1994). *Cultural politics and identity formation in a San Joaquin Valley Hmong community*. Unpublished doctoral dissertation, University of California, Los Angeles, California.

Belenky, M. F., Clinchy, B. M., Goldberger, N. R., & Tarule, J. M. (1986) *Women's ways of knowing: The development of self, voice, and mind*. New York, NY: Basic Books.

Burden, D. S., & Klerman, L. V. (1984, January/February). Teenage parenthood: Factors that lessen economic dependence. *Social Work*, *29*, 11–16.

Center for Cross-Cultural Health. (2000). *Hmong culture: A profile in Minnesota*. Minneapolis, MN: Author.

Cole, P. M., & Tan, P. Z. (2007). Emotion socialization from a cultural perspective. In J. E. Grusec & P. D Hastings (Eds.), *Handbook of socialization* (pp. 516–542). New York: Guildford Press.

Dahl, G. B. (2010). Early teen marriage and future poverty. *Demography*, *47*(3), 689–718.

Dix, T. (1991). The affective organization of parenting: Adaptive and maladaptive processes. *Psychological Bulletin*, *110*, 3–25.

Donnelly, N. (1994). *Changing lives of refugee women*. Seattle, WA: University of Washington Press.

Downing, B. T. (1984). *The Hmong Resettlement Study Site Report: Minneapolis-St. Paul*. Submitted by Northwest Regional Educational Laboratory, Portland, OR to the Office of Refugee Resettlement, Washington, DC.

Dunnigan, T., Onley, D., McNall, M. A., & Spring, M. A. (1996). Hmong. In D. W. Haines (Ed.), *Refugees in America in the 1990s: A reference handbook* (pp. 132–175). New York, NY: Holt, Rinehart and Winston.

Eccles, J. S. (1999). The development of children ages 6–14. *The Future of Children, 9*(2), 30–44.

Erikson, E. (1968). *Identity: Youth and crisis.* New York, NY: Norton.

Folkman, S. (1984). Personal control and stress and coping processes: A theoretical analysis. *Journal of Personality and Social Psychology, 46,* 839–852.

Fontes, L. A. (2005). *Child abuse and culture: Working with diverse families.* New York, NY: Guilford Press.

Glaser, B. G., & Strauss, A. L. (1967). *The discovery of Grounded Theory: Strategies for qualitative research.* Chicago, IL: Aldine Publishing Company.

Greenberg, J., & Cheselka, O. (1995). Relational approaches to psychoanalytical psycho-therapy. In A. S. Gurman & S. B. Messer (Eds.), *Essential psychotherapies: Therapy and practice* (pp. 55–85). New York, NY: Guilford Press.

Hamilton-Merritt, J. (1993). *Tragic mountains: The Hmong, the Americans, and the secret wars for Laos, 1942–1992.* Bloomington, IN: Indiana University Press.

Hein, J. (2006). *Ethnic origins: The adaptation of Cambodian and Hmong refugees in four American cities.* New York, NY: Russell Sage Foundation.

Hutchison, R., & McNall, M. (1994). Early marriage in a Hmong cohort. *Journal of Marriage and the Family, 56,* 579–590.

Koltyk, J. A. (1998). *New pioneers in the heartland: Hmong life in Wisconsin.* Needham Heights, MA: Allyn & Bacon.

Langellier, K. M. (2002). Performing family stories, forming cultural identity: Franco American Memere stories. *Communication Studies, 53,* 56–73.

Larson, R. W., Wilson, S., & Rickman, A. (2009). Globalization, societal change, and adolescence across the world. In R. M. Lerner & L. Steinberg (Eds.), *Handbook of adolescent psychology* (vol. 2, 3rd ed., pp. 590–622). New York, NY: Wiley.

Lee, R. M., Jung, K. R., Su, J. C., Train, A. G. T. T., & Bahrassa, N. E. (2009). The family life and adjustment of Hmong American sons and daughters. *Sex Roles, 60,* 549–558.

Lee, S. J. (1997). The road to college: Hmong American women's pursuit of higher education. *Harvard Educational Review, 67*(4), 803–827.

Lee, S. C., Xiong, Z. B., & Yuen, F. K. O. (2006). Explaining early marriage in the Hmong American community. In H. Holgate, R. Evans, & F. K. Yuen (Eds.), *Teen pregnancy and parenthood: Global perspectives, issues, and interventions* (pp. 25–37). London, Great Britain: Taylor & Francis.

Lo, K. (2002). *Across the ocean: The impact of immigration on Hmong women.* Unpublished master's thesis. University of Wisconsin, Menomonie, Wisconsin.

McNall, M., Dunnigan, T., & Mortimer, J. T. (1994, March). The educational achievement of the St. Paul Hmong. *Anthropology & Education Quarterly, 25*(1), 44–65.

Meschke, L. L. (2003). The Lao Family SPRANS Assessment Project. Unpublished report. St. Paul, MN.

Mischel W. (1973) Towards a cognitive, social learning reconception of personality. *Psychological Review, 80,* 252–283.

Minnesota State Legislature. (2006a). S.F. No 2043 Hmong marriage. Retrieved from http://www.senate.leg.state.mn.us/departments/scr/billsumm/summary_display.php?ls=84&session=regular&body=Senate&billtype=SF&billnumber=2403&ss_year=0

Minnesota State Legislature. (2006b). HF 3674 Hmong marriage. Retrieved from http://www.house.leg.state.mn.us/hrd/bs/84/HF3674.html

Minnesota State Legislature. (2006c). Hmong cultural marriages. Retrieved from http://www.house.leg.state.mn.us/hrd/bs/84/HF3674.html

Moore, K. A., Myers, D. E., Morrison, D. R., Nord, C. W., Brown, B., & Edmonston, B. (1993). Age at first childbirth and later poverty. *Journal of Research on Adolescence, 3,* 393–422.

Moua, T. (2003). The Hmong culture: Kinship, marriage, and family systems [Electronic version]. Retrieved from http://www.uwstout.edu/lib/thesis/2003/2003mouat.pdf

National Association of Social Workers. (2008). *Code of Ethics of the National Association of Social Workers.* Washington, DC: Author.

Ngo, B. (2002). Contesting "culture": The perspectives of Hmong American female students on early marriage. *Anthropology & Education Quarterly, 22*(2), 163–188.

Pho, T., & Mulvey, A. (2003). South East Asian women in Lowell: Family relations, gender roles, and community concerns. *Frontiers—A Journal of Women's Studies, 24,* 101–132.

Sears, R. R. (1975). Your ancients revisited: A history of child development. In E. M. Hetherington (Ed.), *Review of child development research* (Vol. 5, pp. 1–80). Chicago, IL: University of Chicago Press.

Sharlin, S. A. (1998). The impact of demographic social support and marital context variables on the quality of adolescent marriage. *International Journal of Comparative Sociology, 39*(4), 384–398.

Stevens-Simon, C., & Lowy, R. (1995). Teenage childbearing: An adaptive strategy for the socioeconomically disadvantaged or a strategy for adapting to socioeconomic disadvantage? *Archives of Pediatrics and Adolescent Medicine, 149,* 912–915.

Swartz, T., Lee, J. C., & Mortimer, J. T. (2003). Achievements of first generation Hmong youth: Findings from the Youth Development Study. *CURA Reporter*. University of Minnesota, 15–21.

Symonds, P. V. (2004). *Gender and the cycle of life: Calling in the soul in a Hmong village*. Seattle, WA: University of Washington Press.

Teti, D. M., & Lamb, M. E. (1989). Socioeconomic and marital outcomes of adolescent marriages, adolescent childbirth and their co-occurrence. *Journal of Marriage and the Family*, *51*, 203–212.

Thao, C. T. (1986). Hmong customs on marriage, divorce, and the rights of married women. In B. Johns & D. Strecker (Eds.), *The Hmong world* (pp. 74–97). New Haven, CT: Council on Southeast Asian Studies.

Upchurch, D. M. (1993). Early schooling and childbearing experiences: Implications for postsecondary school attendance. *Journal of Research on Adolescence*, *3*(4), 423–443.

Vang, P. D., & Bogenschutz, M. (2011). The effects of early marriage on the socioeconomic status of Hmong women. *International Migration*. doi: 10.1111/j.1468-2435.2010.00674.x

Vang, P. D., & Bogenschutz, M. (2013). Early marriage and mental health among Hmong women. *Journal of Social Work, 13*, 164–183. doi: 10.1177/1468017311409135

White, M. (2004). *Narrative practice and exotic lives: Resurrecting diversity in everyday life*. Adelaide, S. Australia: Dulwich Centre Publications.

Puerto Rican Intergroup Marriage and Residential Segregation in the U.S.: A Multilevel Analysis of Structural, Cultural, and Economic Factors

Anthony De Jesús

Department of Social Work & Latino Community Practice, University of Saint Joseph, West Hartford, Connecticut, USA

Giovani Burgos

Department of Sociology, Stony Brook University, Stony Brook, New York, USA

Melissa Almenas

Center for Safety and Change, New City, New York, USA

William Velez

Department of Sociology, University of Wisconsin–Milwaukee, Milwaukee, Wisconsin, USA

This study examines intermarriage patterns of Puerto Ricans who reside in the United States (referred to as stateside Puerto Ricans) and discusses the implications of these patterns for practice with this community. Because Puerto Ricans experience higher levels of intermarriage than other Latino groups, an analysis of out-marriage factors for Puerto Ricans yields important considerations for the future of Latino integration within U.S. society.

Our primary focus is on whether residential segregation has an impact on Puerto Rican marriage patterns above and beyond the effects of socioeconomic status (SES) and acculturation, as proposed by numerous theories of assimilation (discussed below). We operationalize integration as out-marriage to non-Hispanic Whites (i.e., Whites).

The macro-structural conditions, such as segregation, that shape the incorporation of Puerto Ricans into mainstream society are poorly understood. Drawing on classic and contemporary theories of immigrant *and* minority incorporation, we ask whether residential segregation impacts the likelihood that Puerto Ricans will marry other Puerto Ricans, other Latinos, and Blacks, relative to the likelihood that they will marry Whites. Individual-level data from the American Community Survey is merged with data from the U.S. Census (SF-1 & SF-2) at the county level. Multinomial logistic regression and hierarchical linear modeling results reveal that segregation continues to be a powerful social characteristic of place that affects intermarriage and the incorporation of Puerto Ricans in ways that call into question cultural and over-individualized explanations of life chances.

This study examines intermarriage patterns of Puerto Ricans who reside in the United States (referred to as stateside Puerto Ricans) and discusses the implications of these patterns for practice with this community. Our primary focus is on whether residential segregation has an impact on Puerto Rican marriage patterns above and beyond the effects of SES and acculturation, as proposed by numerous theories of assimilation (discussed below). The study of intermarriage provides an opportunity to explore larger issues of racial and ethnic integration within the United States because Puerto Ricans are U.S. citizens by birth with a long accelerating migration pattern to the continental United States (Vélez & Burgos, 2010). Additionally, the study of Puerto Rican intermarriage provides a useful case study of the ways in which out-marriage to members of the dominant group may be influenced by cultural, economic, and structural forces. Analysis of the marriage patterns of stateside Puerto Ricans provides an important understanding of the ways in which Puerto Ricans are adapting to economic and cultural forces on the mainland through their marriage choices. Interpreted through classical and contemporary theories on marriage and assimilation and the racialized place inequality framework advanced by Burgos & Rivera (2012), this article identifies the most salient forces impacting Puerto Ricans' marriage patterns and discusses the implications of these findings for social work practice with Puerto Ricans.

Demographic shifts within the U.S. population (i.e., dramatic increases in the number of Latinos and other racialized minorities) and long-standing racial inequalities complicate established assimilation narratives, particularly those characterized by the "melting pot" metaphor (see Scott & Marshall, 2009). This enduring metaphor conveys the assumption that new immigrant groups will replace their cultural and linguistic practices with those of the dominant "American culture" over the course of a few generations. *Classic spatial assimilation theory* (Alba & Nee, 2002) particularly holds that immigrant groups become increasingly integrated with the dominant group as they acquire levels of human capital, group culture, and attitudes that characterize the dominant group. (Iceland & Nelson, 2010). Thus, much like their White European peers did in the nineteenth and twentieth centuries (see Steinberg, 1981), this theory predicts that, over time, racialized minorities (e.g., Blacks, Latinos, Asians) will assimilate (i.e., learn English, become college educated, acquire the lifestyles and behavioral patterns of the dominant groups, amass economic resources) and integrate (e.g., marry and live in the same neighborhoods) with the dominant group (i.e., White protestants of European descent). The assimilation process nears completion when groups move out of racial/ethnic enclaves in the inner city (i.e., ghettoes and barrios) and into integrated residential areas with Whites, most likely in the suburbs (Grosfoguel & Georas, 2000).

Exogamy, the practice of minority group individuals marrying persons of the dominant culture, has been a longstanding indicator of assimilation for minority groups that may emphasize maintenance of linguistic and cultural ties through ethnic endogamy (Fu, 2007). In fact, Gordon (1964) argued that intermarriage was the final stage in the assimilation process and that high rates of intermarriage were indicative of diminished levels of social distance, racism, and discrimination in American society. Clearly, marriage between majority and minority groups is viewed as an essential component of the assimilation process and is expected to aid minorities to make the successful transition to full social integration and also, to significantly aid minorities to reach the American dream of upward economic and social mobility. Thus, classic spatial assimilation theory predicts that minorities of higher SES, and those with greater levels of acculturation will have greater rates of intermarriage with the dominant group than minorities of lower SES and those who are less acculturated to the dominant group.

Critics of assimilation theories contend that such theories do not take into account the political economy of race relations and that such theories incorrectly assume that the experiences of White Europeans in the last two centuries are similar, or even identical to, the experiences of Black Americans and other racialized minorities, such as Puerto Ricans. More specifically, critical race theorists and scholars writing from the vantage point of the *place stratification framework* note that the United States remains a highly stratified society along racial and ethnic lines because racism and discrimination continue to limit the life chances of racialized minorities (McKee, 1993; Leiman, 2010; Blauner, 2001). In the United States, structural racism and discrimination are phenotypically and color-based so that individuals of Black phenotype and/or dark skin have more experiences with discrimination in the housing and labor market than Whites and their lighter skin peers (Burton, Bonilla-Silva, Ray, Buckelew, & Freeman, 2010). Critical and place stratification scholars acknowledge that although White Europeans experienced ethnic based discrimination, their color and phenotype allowed them to melt into the larger pot of whiteness as they became more acculturated and became residentially integrated with the dominant White group.

In contrast, race and color-based discrimination in the housing and rental markets has stalled the spatial assimilation process for African Americans and Puerto Ricans, as reflected by high levels of segregation between these two groups from Whites. As Burgos and Rivera (2012) recently point out, residential segregation between Whites and Puerto Ricans/African Americans results from systemic acts of discrimination by Whites against minorities in the housing and rental market. These acts of discrimination prevent minorities from sharing residential spaces with dominant groups. As a result, the United States remains a divided society, with Whites more likely to live in resource-rich neighborhoods while African Americans and Puerto Ricans are more likely to live in economically disadvantaged communities (Carr & Kutty, 2008a; Massey & Denton, 1993). For instance, between the years 1980 and 2000, Latinos experienced overall increases in segregation, and Puerto Ricans are the second most segregated minority group after African Americans (Wilkes & Iceland, 2004; Reardon et al., 2009). Among Latinos, stateside Puerto Ricans have been, and continue to be, the most highly segregated ethnic group in the United States (Vargas-Ramos, 2006; Vélez & Burgos, 2010). Fair housing advocates also maintain that segregation is a direct result of systemic acts of discrimination against racialized minorities in the housing market (Carr & Kutty, 2008a) and note that a central policy concern is that racialized minorities disproportionately bear the brunt of limited life chances associated with segregation, such as low SES, poor health, high levels of stress, crime and delinquency, teen pregnancy, high school dropout, and other problems that limit the chances of upward mobility (Acevedo-Garcia & Osypuk, 2008).

The problem, for the purposes of this paper, is that these high levels of segregation are self-reinforcing and threaten racial and ethnic integration. Thus, according to the place stratification framework, Puerto Ricans living in counties with high levels of White/Puerto Rican segregation are expected to be less integrated with Whites or to have lower levels of inter-marriage with Whites than Puerto Ricans living in less segregated counties.

Although the study of intergroup marriage is central to our understanding of social integration, the effects that structural factors such as residential segregation have on intermarriage between Whites and Puerto Ricans are largely unexplored. To date, little is known about the effects that residential segregation has on Puerto Rican marriage patterns above and beyond the effects proposed by classic spatial assimilation theory, such as SES (i.e., income, education, wealth, occupational prestige, poverty status) and levels of acculturation (e.g., generational status, English proficiency).

BACKGROUND

Annexed by the United States in 1898 as a spoil of the Spanish American War, Puerto Rico has endured as a territory of the United States creating the conditions for longstanding migration between the island and the mainland United States—a pattern that accelerated in the post-WW II period (Collazo, Ryan, & Bauman, 2010; Duany, 2002). The Jones Act of 1917 made Puerto Ricans U.S. citizens, a fact that has facilitated circular migration in response to labor market forces on the mainland for the second half of the twentieth century. While New York City was the primary destination for many early migrants, other northeastern and Midwestern communities experienced growth of their Puerto Rican populations and the establishment of Puerto Rican enclaves.

The *vaiven* (coming and going) of migration has profoundly affected Puerto Rican identity and integration with the dominant group. Scholars have argued that the more than 8 million Puerto Ricans living on the island and the mainland United States constitute an *ethnonation* that extends itself across political and cultural borders as Puerto Ricans have renegotiated shifts in their identities from territorially bounded ones, to affective and cultural identities (Aranda, 2006; Grosfoguel & Georas, 2000). While Puerto Ricans on the island have maintained a distinct Latin American national identity, their ties to *Nuyorican* and *Diasporican* relatives are shaped in response to local conditions of stateside Puerto Ricans and the relationship of those communities to economic opportunity, or the lack thereof. Such revolving migration patterns and strong ethnic identity put into question the canonical notion of assimilation or the assumption that Puerto Ricans will follow the "the gradual, uniform process of upward mobility and incorporation into society's mainstream" that characterized the experience of early European immigrants (see Portes, Fernández-Kelly, & Haller, 2005, p. 1002).

Still, stateside Puerto Ricans have fought hard to be incorporated into mainstream society and have long asserted their political rights in response to discrimination and exclusion within U.S. institutions. This was especially evident during the civil rights era where Puerto Ricans in New York City organized for community control of schools in coalition with African Americans and successfully filed a law suit to establish bilingual education in New York City schools (De Jesús & Perez, 2009). Using activism and protest to address oppressive conditions during this period, the Young Lords Party occupied public institutions as a way to highlight the ways in which Puerto Ricans and other communities were being denied services and excluded from institutions that facilitated upward mobility (Enck-Wanzer, 2010; Melendez & Visser, 2011). A number of national and regional organizations and institutions were founded during the civil rights period that served Puerto Ricans and other Latino communities today. Among the most prominent are Aspira of America, the National Congress of Puerto Rican Rights, and the Center for Puerto Rican Studies at Hunter College (Totti & Matos Rodriguez, 2009). Despite many advances, a large segment of this community continues to experience challenges in regard to educational attainment, labor force participation, and full participatory integration with mainstream society (De Jesús & Vásquez, 2005; Melendez & Visser, 2011).

In 2010, there were significant numbers of Puerto Ricans residing in eight sun-belt states like Florida, which replaced rust-belt states in the northeast and Midwest as the preferred destination of Puerto Rican migrants. Between 2000 and 2006, 6 of the 10 counties with the fastest Puerto Rican growth were found in Florida (Vélez & Burgos, 2010). The Puerto Rican population in the United States is increasingly bifurcated in terms of income and housing. Large numbers remain in impoverished and segregated neighborhoods while still others are enjoying relatively higher incomes and moving to more affluent suburbs. For example, in 2006, Puerto Ricans in Hartford (Connecticut) were earning an average wage of only $24,000, while their counterparts in Nassau County (New York) were earning an average wage close to $61,000. It appears, then, that Puerto Ricans with higher levels of education and holding more prestigious jobs are earning good salaries when they live in more integrated counties (Vélez & Burgos, 2010). In a more recent study, Burgos and Rivera (2012) found that Puerto Ricans living in counties where they were highly segregated from Whites had higher rates of disability than Puerto Ricans living in counties where they were more integrated with Whites. Thus, segregation systematically structures the prospects of Puerto Ricans. These findings show that segregation affects Puerto Rican life chances, at least in terms of SES and disability, and they also suggest that segregation might be related to Puerto Rican's level of social integration and patterns of intermarriage.

If we assume these more successful Puerto Ricans are following the traditional assimilation processes experienced by prior European immigrants, then Puerto Rican's out-marriage to Whites should be higher in counties where they are more residentially integrated with the dominant group. Unfortunately, little is known about how segregation shapes the marriage patterns between Puerto Ricans and other groups. Even less is known about how segregation affects Puerto Rican marriage patterns above and beyond the effects of other individual-level predictors of interracial marriage.

To examine whether segregation affects patterns of interracial and intergroup marriage among Puerto Ricans, we draw on the *Racialized Place Inequality Framework* recently developed by Burgos and Rivera (2012). One of our central concerns is whether segregation is related to inter-marriage above and beyond the effects of other know correlates of exogamy, such as socioeconomic status and acculturation (e.g., Davis, 1941; Kalmijn, 1998; Merton, 1941).

RACIALIZED PLACE INEQUALITY FRAMEWORK

The racialized place inequality framework (RPIF) introduced by Burgos & Rivera (2012), which draws on insights of place stratification scholars, is based on the premise that residential segregation is a direct result of discrimination in the rental and housing markets against racial minorities, including African Americans and Puerto Ricans. For instance, segregation has been fueled by anti-miscegenation laws that were "Aimed at preserving racial purity of the white race [and preventing] interracial couples from marrying and producing legitimate racially mixed children [since such children] would destabilize a system of racial apartheid [that preserved] white privilege and supremacy" (Oh, 2005, pp. 1320–1321). These laws were purposely designed to preserve social and geographical boundaries between Blacks and Whites and to sustain a system of separate and unequal institutions whose effects are still with us today in the form of residential segregation and its negative consequences.

Other discriminatory practices that have also created separate and unequal residential areas between Puerto Ricans/Blacks and Whites include the building of housing projects in poor urban communities by the federal government, the passing of building codes by local governments that limit the number of people who can live in an apartment and that prohibit the building of multi-unit dwellings, the *redlining* by banks of predominantly minority areas on a map for the sole purpose of denying mortgages to minorities in those communities, the higher denial rates by mortgage insurance companies to minorities that makes owning a home in more expensive/exclusive neighborhoods unlikely, the *steering* by real estate agents of minorities away from White neighborhoods, the refusal of landlords in White neighborhoods to rent to minorities and to individuals with Section 8 vouchers, and Whites' strong preferences to live in all-White communities, including leaving neighborhoods that are "turning" and becoming more racially and ethnically diverse—a process known as *White flight* (see Miller, Vandome, & McBrewster, 2009; U.S. Housing Scholars & Research and Advocacy Organizations, 2008; Carr & Kutty, 2008a; Roscigno, Karafin, & Tester, 2009).

Housing discrimination practices such as these, among others, have led to some powerful conclusions by place stratification scholars about the social detriments that result from segregation. For instance, Williams and Collins (2001, p. 404) argue that segregation is a direct result of systemic acts of housing discrimination that "protect Whites from interaction with Blacks" and other minorities. Rugh and Massey (2010, p. 630) indicate that segregation "concentrates the effects of any economic downturn spatially . . . and hit Black and Hispanic neighborhoods with particular force." Carr and Kutty (2008b, p. 1) maintain that "denial of access to housing is arguably the single most powerful tool to undermine and marginalize the upward mobility of people." Perhaps not surprisingly, place stratification scholars have referred to residential segregation as the "lynchpin of American race relations" (Bobo & Zubrinsky, 1996).

These statements are not surprising given that residential segregation significantly limits the life chances of African Americans and Puerto Ricans. As captured by the RPIF that appears in Figure 1, segregation is a macro-level characteristic of place (metropolitan area, state, county) that sets into motion a series of disadvantages at the meso-level, such as economically disadvantage neighborhoods with high crime rates, dilapidated housing, poorly built environment, lack of access to quality health care, and toxic environments. In turn, these meso-level conditions concentrate disadvantages at the micro-individual level including low SES, high levels of stress/discrimination, and lack of social integration. While the model was developed to study health disparities, it also captures the effects that segregation has on social integration, including network ties, and social support. We consider interracial marriages an indicator of social integration. This framework is particularly relevant for this analysis of intermarriage as Puerto Ricans are the most highly segregated Latino ethnic group in the United States (Massey & Denton, 1993; Vargas-Ramos, 2006; Vélez & Burgos, 2010). As the negative consequences of segregation converge in minority communities, the *racialization of place* may also play a considerable role in the marriage patterns of Puerto Ricans.

There is great variation in terms of segregation in the areas where Puerto Ricans live. The northeastern region of the United States and major cities such as New York were the primary destination for the first wave of Puerto Rican migrants leading to the establishment of well-known ethnic enclaves such as *El Barrio* in Manhattan. The New York metropolitan area and the neighborhoods where Puerto Ricans live were also characterized by residential segregation and concentrated poverty. However, during the early twenty-first century, Puerto Rican migration patterns have shifted considerably with many Puerto Ricans leaving urban areas for the suburbs and new sun-belt destinations such as Central Florida (Torres, Marzán, & Luecke, 2008; Silver, 2010; Duany, 2010). As a result, the combination of more educated Puerto Rican workers and the availability of affordable housing in suburban neighborhoods may facilitate the conditions for more contact with other ethnic groups and, thus, higher levels of exogamy. The migration from the island to mainland and back, known as circular migration, as well as between urban and suburban areas, further diversifies the geographic communities and marriage markets in which Puerto Ricans will seek a partner. In addition to segregation, the RPIF also acknowledges that other structural conditions can affect the marriage patterns of Puerto Ricans including group size and economic conditions at the macro-level (Christensen, 2011). Although marriage is often thought about as related to personal choice, structural conditions profoundly influence the social conditions under which one chooses a marriage partner.

THEORIES OF INTERMARRIAGE

A number of theories related to intermarriage and immigrant incorporation provide potential explanations for Puerto Rican marriage patterns. S*tatus-case exchange theory* (Merton, 1941; Davis, 1941) was advanced to describe interracial marriages in the United States during a period when Jim Crow laws were still in effect. Merton and Davis argued that Black men who could achieve higher SES than Black women were more likely to marry White women than Black women were to marry White men. They proposed that the increase in socioeconomic status for Black men offset their racial status in attracting White female spouses (Jacobs & Labov, 2002; Kincannon, 2010). Status class exchange theory would therefore expect higher-SES Puerto Ricans to marry Whites to a greater degree than their lower-SES peers. Further, due to shifting gender roles, and high incarceration rates among Puerto Rican men, Puerto Rican women have been able to attain higher education and SES levels than their male counterparts (Enchautegui & Freeman, 2006). As a result, status-caste exchange theory would predict that Puerto Rican women are more likely partners for White men.

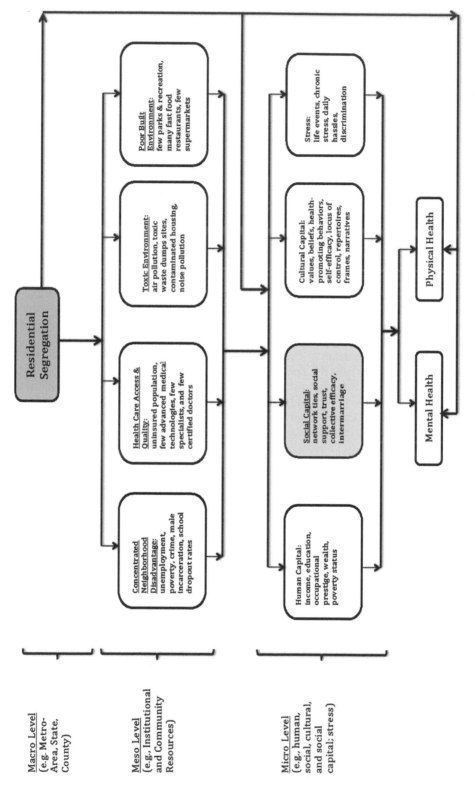

FIGURE 1   The racialized place inequality framework: How segregation affects integration.

Gordon's (1964) seminal work on assimilation introduced intermarriage as an indicator of assimilation (see also Alba & Nee, 2002; Rumbaut, 1997). Gordon however, prematurely regarded intermarriage as the last stage of assimilation between Anglo Americans and ethnic groups in American society and, thus, did not fully capture the complexity of marriage in a multiracial/multicultural society (Qian and Lichter, 2001).[1] Classic assimilation theory highlights the importance of linguistic assimilation that allows for greater group contact and interaction. English proficiency is a crucial determinant of Latino mobility patterns as it allows Latinos to enter majority-dominant neighborhoods and possibly obtain better jobs (Alba & Nee, 1997). The literature shows that island-born and first-generation Puerto Ricans have higher rates of endogamy than mainland-born and later-generation Puerto Ricans (Aquino, 2011; Lichter, Carmalt, & Qian, 2011). Thus, we expect Puerto Ricans born in the United States and those who have been in the United States longer will be more likely to marry Whites than Puerto Ricans born in Puerto Rico or individuals who have fewer years living in the United States. There is also strong evidence that racial identification will predict out-marriage, as Puerto Ricans who identify as Black are 16 times more likely to marry a Black American than a White American (Aquino, 2011). Thus, according to classic assimilation models such as Gordon's, we expect Puerto Ricans who are more acculturated (i.e., speak English, born in the United States, lived in the United States the longest) to have higher rates of intermarriage to Whites than Puerto Ricans with lower levels of acculturation.

Building on Gordon's work, Portes and Zhou (1993) introduced *segmented assimilation theory*, which places SES, particularly education, at the center of immigrant incorporation and integration and incorporated patterns of second-wave immigration from Latin America, the Caribbean, Africa, and some parts of Asia. Segmented assimilation theory outlines three possible outcomes for an immigrant group: (1) traditional assimilation patterns over at least three generations leading to upward collective mobility (e.g., "out of the barrio"); (2) downward mobility by failing (or refusing) to adopt cultural ways of the dominant group and by unsuccessfully competing in the mainstream economy; or (3) upward mobility by living and working in ethnically homogeneous immigrant communities (Portes & Rumbaut, 2001). Downward assimilation and ethnic enclaves can be viewed as both the result of individual-level characteristics (linguistic and socioeconomic homogamy), which collectively result in a particular residential arrangement that affects the probability of out-marriage for its inhabitants. Thus, according to segmented assimilation theory, more educated Puerto Ricans will be more likely to marry Whites compared to less educated Puerto Ricans.

RESEARCH QUESTIONS

We are primarily interested in the effects that residential segregation has on Puerto Rican marriage patterns and in examining the robustness of such a relationship. In other words, does the relationship between segregation and intermarriage hold when controlling for other individual level characteristics that are related to intermarriage, such as SES, measures of acculturation, and other demographic factors including race and gender? The literature on interracial marriages shows that higher-SES (e.g., education) Latinos are more likely to marry Whites than their lower-SES peers (Kincannon, 2010; Qian & Lichter, 2007). Both classic spatial assimilation theory (Alba & Nee, 1997, 2002) and segmented assimilation theory (Portes & Rumbaut, 2001; Portes et al., 2005) suggest that more acculturated minorities, or those who speak English and have been in the United States for longer periods of time are more likely to integrate with the dominant group than their less acculturated counterparts (Lichter et al., 2011). The literature also shows that island-born and first-generation Puerto Ricans and Latino have higher rates of endogamy than mainland-born and later-generation Puerto Ricans and Latinos (Aquino, 2011; Lichter et al., 2011). In terms of gender, there is some work showing that rates of out-marriage to Whites is higher among Puerto Rican and Latina Women than among Puerto Rican and Latino men (Qian & Lichter, 2001; Jacobs & Labov, 2002; Aquino, 2011). There is also strong evidence that racial identification will predict exogamy, as Puerto Ricans who identify as Black are 16 times more likely to marry a Black American than a White American (Aquino, 2011). Thus, it is important to control for these important individual-level characteristics when evaluation the effects of segregation on intermarriage.

This study poses the following research questions:

1. Do micro-level measures of acculturation (language, time in United States), SES (occupational prestige, education, income, poverty), and demographic factors (race, gender) affect the likelihood of Puerto Rican out-marriage, particularly marriage to Whites?
2. How do macro-structural factors, measured by segregation, social disorganization, and economic disadvantage variables, affect the likelihood of Puerto Rican out-marriage, particularly marriage to Whites?
3. Does the relationship between segregation and intermarriage, if any, hold when controlling for acculturation, SES, and basic demographic factors?

DATA AND METHODS

Data

This paper merges individual-level data from the 2005–2009 Integrated Public Use Micro-Data Samples (IPUMS) with county-level data from 2000 U.S. Census Summary Files 1 and 3. The combined data are used for the multilevel analyses where individuals are nested within counties. IPUMS is a nationally representative sample that was extracted from the yearly American Community Survey (ACS). The ACS is a monthly rolling sample of household and individuals within those households and was designed to approximate and ultimately replace estimates from the U.S. Decennial Census long form. The primary goal of the ACS is to provide both policy makers and researchers with data on the social and economic well-being of the population, such as occupational prestige, income, education, poverty, disability status, family composition, migration, and race/ethnic background on a timely basis. All person-level variables (i.e., level-1 variables in the hierarchical linear model framework [HLM] context) in this study came from the ACS IPUMS data (overall response rate is 97.5). The 5% sample of the IPUMS combines data from the yearly 1% samples that were collected from 2005 to 2009. Aside from the decennial Census, these data encompass one of the largest samples of Puerto Ricans in the United States. Complete descriptions of the complex cluster-sample design of ACS IPUMS data have been widely disseminated elsewhere (Ruggles et al., 2010; U.S. Census Bureau, 2006).

Structural or level-two variables at the county level come from two other data sets: 2000 Census Summary File 1 (SF 1) and Summary File 3 (SF 3). Whereas SF 1, which is based on the Census 2000 Short-Form, contains 100%-data on population characteristics such as age, gender, ethnicity, race, household relationships, family composition, and other basic demographic factors (U.S. Census Bureau, 2001a), SF 3 contains a more extensive list of variables and is based on sample (i.e., not a complete count) data (U.S. Census Bureau, 2001b). Estimates from these summary files can also be produced for the whole nation down to the block level.

To combine these data, we first geo-coded the IPUMS data and assigned a census county code to each respondent. The IPUMS data were then merged with SF 1 and SF 3 by county code. For the level-1 analyses, we created two samples. First, we analyzed these IPUMS data for all Puerto Ricans in the United States ($N = 1,050,357$, weighted count). Second, for the multilevel analyses, we restricted the sample to Puerto Ricans living in 72 U.S. counties. This was a data-driven restriction, given the current interest in counties with large numbers of Puerto Ricans, methodological concerns about counties having large numbers of individuals at level one in a multi-level context to produce reliable estimates (Raudenbush & Bryk, 2002) and issues about the size of the minority population when constructing segregation indices (Wilkes & Iceland, 2004, p. 24). Therefore, counties that had 1,000 or more Puerto Ricans (estimated from SF 1) were selected for the multilevel analyses. These criteria resulted in a large sample of Puerto Ricans ($N = 31,746$, un-weighted) living in 72 different counties throughout the United States—or about 440 Puerto Ricans per county. Puerto Ricans living in these 72 counties vary widely on a wide range of social and economic characteristics. To date, this is the largest and most geographically varied multilevel study on segregation and inter-group marriage among Puerto Ricans in the United States.

Individual Level-1 Variables from 2005–2009 IPUMS

Dependent Variable

For type of intergroup marriage, we created a nominal variable of the racial and ethnic background of the couple of each Puerto Rican in our sample. As summarized in Table 1, 54% of Puerto Ricans are married to other Puerto Ricans. About 15% of Puerto Ricans are married to other Latinos, and almost a fourth (23%) of Puerto Ricans are married to non-Latino Whites. The proportion of Puerto Ricans married to African Americans (3%) and individuals from some other background (2%) is much lower, by comparison. This nominal variable includes five categories, including Puerto Ricans who are married to 1 = *other Puerto Ricans*, 2 = *other Latinos*, 3 = *Whites*, 4 = *African Americans*, and 5 = *individuals of another race/ethnicity*. Descriptive statistics for all dependent and independent variables appear in Table 1.

Independent Variables

Our models control for basic demographic variables including *age* in years as of the last birthday, dummies for *gender* (1 = male, 0 = female), and dummies for *race* (Black Puerto Rican, mixed Puerto Rican, and White Puerto Rican as the reference category). SES indicators include respondents' total personal *income* (logged); *educational attainment* (e.g., 1 = no school completed, 5 = fifth–eighth grade, 9 = ninth–twelfth grade, no diploma, 10 = high school graduate, or GED, 14 = bachelor's degrees, 17 = doctorate degree); *wealth* (1 = *owns home*, 0 = *rents and/or does not own home*); and Duncan's (1961) index of *occupational prestige* that ranges from low to high, and *poverty status* (1 = at or below poverty threshold ... 5 = 500% or more above poverty threshold). *Acculturation* is indexed with three variables: whether the respondents were *born in the United States* (1 = *born in the United States*, 0 = *born elsewhere*); *the number of years respondents have lived in the United States*; and whether *English is the primary language spoken at home* (1 = *English is primary language spoken*, 0 = *Spanish and/or some other language spoken*).

County Level-2 Variables

As regards residential segregation, the *isolation index* measures the extent to which Puerto Ricans are exposed to other Puerto Ricans and ranges from 0 (Puerto Ricans are completely integrated with Whites) to 1 (Puerto Ricans are completely isolated from Whites). Formally:

$$I = \sum_{i}^{n} \left[\left(\frac{pr_i}{PR} \right) \left(\frac{w_i}{t_i} \right) \right]$$

TABLE 1

Descriptive Statistics for Selected Variables from 2005–2009 Integrated Public Use
Microdata Series (IPUMS), $N = 1,050,357$

Variables	Mean	S.E.	Minimum	Maximum
Individual Level-1 Variables				
Dependent Variable: Type of Puerto Rican Inter-Group Marriage				
Puerto Rican Married to Other Puerto Rican = 1 (P)	0.548	—	—	—
Puerto Rican Married to Other Latino = 2 (O)	0.153	—	—	—
Puerto Rican Married to Non-Latino White = 3 (W)	0.231	—	—	—
Puerto Rican Married to Non-Latino Black = 4 (B)	0.038	—	—	—
Puerto Rican Married to Some Other Race = 5 (R)	0.028	—	—	—
Demographic Variables:				
Age	45.755	0.082	15.000	95.000
Male (1 = male, 0 = female)	0.521	0.002	0.000	1.000
Black (1 = Black, 0 = White or Mixed)	0.035	0.001	0.000	1.000
White (1 = White, 0 = Black or Mixed)	0.587	0.003	0.000	1.000
Mixed (1 = Mixed, 0 = Black or White)	0.378	0.003	0.000	1.000
Economic Variables:				
Total personal income (logged)	10.955	0.006	0.000	14.094
Education (1 = no high school ... 17 = Doctoral Deg.)	6.593	0.016	0.000	11.000
Wealth (1 = Owns Home, 0 = Rents Home)	0.645	0.004	0.000	1.000
Occupational Prestige Index	31.844	0.113	0.000	1.000
Above Poverty Threshold (1 = 100, 5 = 500)	3.606	0.009	1.000	5.000
Acculturation Variables:				
Born in the United States (1 = yes, 0 = no)	0.476	0.003	0.000	1.000
Years in Living in the United States	16.079	0.102	0.000	90.000
English Primary Language Spoken	0.228	0.002	0.000	1.000
County Level-2 Variables				
Isolation Index (Puerto Rican/White)	0.113	0.011	0.004	0.376
Percent Puerto Rican (year 2009)	4.962	0.503	0.357	23.473
Social Disorganization				
Concentrated Disadvantage	9.013	0.519	9.013	34.356
Residential Instability	515.322	0.580	515.322	540.264
Ethnic Heterogeneity	0.189	0.019	0.189	0.761
Global Status Index	7.300	0.217	7.300	17.274
Percent Low Service Occupations	2.827	0.343	2.827	20.153
Percent Manufacturing	3.517	0.612	3.517	24.244
Percent Urban	61.090	1.034	61.090	100.000

where pr_i is the total number of Puerto Ricans in census tract i, PR is the total number of Puerto Ricans in a county, t_i is the total population in census tract i, and w_i is the total non-Latino White population in tract i. Unlike dissimilarity indices, exposure indices are sensitive to both the distribution and size of the minority population (Bell, 1954; Lieberson, 1981). Early on, Blau (1977) showed that minorities can be evenly distributed in census tracts throughout a city and still have little exposure to Whites and the resources enjoyed in majority tracts. As such, some scholars argue that exposure indices should be stronger predictors of negative life chances than other indices of segregation, such as the index of dissimilarity (Acevedo-Garcia, Lochner, Osypuk, & V., 2003; Kramer & Hogue, 2009). Because we are interested on the effects of both the size and distribution of the Puerto Rican population, the isolation index is preferred to other segregation indices.

Three measures of social disorganization (i.e., concentrated disadvantage index, ethnic hetero-geneity, and residential instability) are included in the analyses (Sampson & Morenoff, 1997; South & Crowder, 1999). Such measures are incorporated since both social disorganization theory and the place stratification framework predict higher levels of social disorganization to be related with problems such as crime and poor health, among other social ills (Latkin & Curry, 2003). We also expect that Puerto Ricans living in more socially disorganized counties will have less contact with Whites, and also, less likely to marry Whites that Puerto Ricans living in less disorganized counties.

Concentrated disadvantage is in an index consisting of the percent of households making less than $10,000 a year, percent on public assistance, percent below the federal poverty line, percent of adults with no high school diploma, percent unemployed, and percent renting in each county, respectively ($\alpha = .74$). As Kubrin and Stewart (2006) note, measures of concentrated disadvantage are preferable over single-item indicators (e.g., percent poor) since they reflect concentration effects that are more consistent with social disorganization theory and theories of urban disadvantage. *Ethnic heterogeneity* is measured with the Herfindahl index of diversity (2000; Rose, 2000). As shown in Table 1, heterogeneity ranges from .18 to .76 with higher values indicating higher levels of ethnic/racial heterogeneity in a county. *Residential instability* was measured by a standardized four-item index (i.e., percent occupied housing units moved into, year householder moved into unit, percent living in different house/county in 1995, and percent living in different house in 1995), with a high internal consistency ($\alpha = .79$). Larger values represent higher levels of residential instability.

County level controls include percent Puerto Rican in 2009 (calculated from the 2005–2009 5% IPUMS), percent employed in low service occupations, percent employed in manufacturing, and percent urban (from SF 3). Drawing on the work of Baird and colleagues (2008), our *global status index* is a scale ($\alpha = .81$) that ranges from low to high in term of the relative strength of the county in global business and financial sectors. The following four items load on a common factor: (1) percent of employees who work in the business sector, (2) percent of labor force in executive administrative, or managerial occupations, (3) percentage of employee earnings in the county from the finance, insurance, and real estate industry (FIRE), and (4) the natural log of the working age population.

In sum, controlling for these important social and economic conditions allows for a more nuanced assessment of the relationship between segregation and Puerto Rican marriage patterns and the robustness of such a relationship.

METHOD AND ANALYTIC STRATEGY

The multivariate analyses in this paper are conducted using hierarchical linear models with the statistical package MPlus 6.12 (2010). As McArdle and Hamagami (1996, p. 89) note, multi-level models have become increasingly popular over the years because they provide a way of dealing with the complexities of "clustered" or "nested" data—such as individuals in counties, neighborhoods, schools and households. Such nesting of individuals within larger social units represents a hierarchical structure where individuals—referred to as level-1 in the hierarchical linear model framework (HLM)—are clustered/found within counties or level-2 units (Raudenbush & Bryk, 2002). This technique has several advantages over traditional methods such as ordinary least square regression where individual-level and county level-variables are included in the same regression equation. HLM allows the analyst to model the dependence of observations within counties, partial out the error variance at level-1 and level-2, and simultaneously model the effects of county level-2 variables separately from the effects of level-1 covariates (Goldstein, 2010; Muthén & Satorra, 1995). With nested data, multi-level modeling produces more reliable and less biased estimates than those generated by traditional single-level regression approaches.

The individual-level 1 model used in this paper takes the following form:

$$\eta_{ij} = \beta_{0j} + \sum_q \beta_q X_{qij} + \varepsilon_{ij}, \tag{1}$$

where η_{ij} is the log-odds of the estimated risk of Puerto Rican individual i in county j being married to other groups (i.e., 1 = *another Puerto Rican*, 2 = *other Latino/a*, 3 = *Whites*, 4 = *Blacks*, 5 = *individuals from some other racial/ethnic group*), β_{0j} is the intercept, X_{ij} is the score of independent variable q (e.g., age, income etc.), and β_q is the regression coefficient associated with variable q.

In the multilevel and multinomial models that we use in this study, we are able to calculate the odds and probability of different marriage combinations (see Hosmer & Lemeshow, 2000). For instance, what is the likelihood that a Puerto Rican individual marries a White individual, or some other group, given their social class, levels of acculturation, and structural conditions of the counties where Puerto Ricans reside?

At level-2, the means as outcome model estimates the average log-odds of inter-group marriage as a predicted by isolation and other county level variables:

$$\beta_{0j} = \gamma_{00} + \gamma_{01}W_{1j} + \gamma_{02}W_{2j} + \gamma_{03}W_{3j} + \ldots \gamma_{0k}W_{kj} + u_{0j}, \tag{2}$$

where γ_{00} is the grand mean, $\gamma_{0k}W_{kj}$ capture the effects of county level variables (isolation, social disorganization, controls) on the risk of out-marriage, say, Whites, and u_{0j} is a county-level random error term. To aid with interpretation, the log of the odds of out-marriage can be converted to odds ratios by exponentiating each logit coefficient (e.g., (exp[isolation]) that is produced by the statistical package, and converting each logit to a probability with a simple transformation [e.g., $1/1 + e^{-(isolation)}$]. These transformations allows for simple interpretation of regression parameters, as shown below (see Long, 1997; Cheong & Raudenbush, 2000).

ANALYTIC PLAN

In Table 1, summary statistics are presented for all individual level-1 variables and county level-2 variables. Table 2 shows multinomial logistic regression coefficients to examine the effects that demographic, class, and acculturation variables have on out-group marriage rates. These analyses are conducted at the individual level-1. The first model in Table 2 captures the odds that Puerto Rican respondents are married to other Puerto Ricans relative to being married to a White person, which is the reference category for all models. The third column in Table 2 captures the odds that Puerto Ricans are married to other Latinos, relative to being married to Whites. The fourth and fifth columns capture the odds that Puerto Ricans are married to African Americans or individuals from some other racial/ethnic background, respectively. To gain a better and more intuitive appreciation of the findings, Table 3 discusses the results in terms of probabilities. Figures 1–3 provide a visual representation of each kind of out-marriage, and how demographic, class, and acculturation variables affect such marriage patterns. In Table 4, results from a multilevel-multinomial regression are presented to gauge how county level variables affect Puerto Rican out-marriage patterns.

TABLE 2

Multinomial Logistic Regression Predicting Marriage to Whites for Puerto Ricans in the United States (Odds Ratios)

Variables	Puerto Rican Married to Puerto Rican (P)	Puerto Rican Married to Other Latino (O)	Puerto Rican Married to Black (B)	Puerto Rican Married to Other Race (R)
Demographic Variables:				
Age	1.023**	0.993**	0.995	1.003
Male (1 = male, 0 = female)	0.930**	1.131**	0.488**	1.218**
White Puerto Rican[R]	—	—	—	—
Black Puerto Rican	2.268**	1.759**	40.569**	4.192**
Mixed Puerto Rican	1.525**	1.458**	4.081**	4.805**
Economic Variables:				
Total personal income (logged)	0.967	1.008	0.975	1.228*
Education	0.861**	0.895**	0.904**	0.997
Wealth (1 = owns home)	0.607**	0.627**	0.542**	0.606**
Occupational Prestige Index	0.997**	1.001	1.005**	1.002
Above Poverty Threshold	0.869**	0.881**	0.966	0.872**
Acculturation Variables:				
Born in the United States (1 = yes)	0.288**	0.503**	1.676**	1.016
Years in Living in the United States	0.973**	0.988**	1.002	0.992*
English Primary Language Spoken	0.133**	0.172**	0.598**	0.813**
Intercept	39.840**	9.426**	0.377	0.013*

Note. P = odds of a Puerto Rican marrying another Puerto Rican *relative* to *Whites*; B = Odds of a Puerto Rican marrying a Black person relative to marrying a White person, and so on.

[R]Reference category.

*$p < .05$. **$p < .01$.

TABLE 3

Probability that a Puerto Rican Individual Marries a White Person from Multinomial Logistic Regression Model

Individual Level-1 Variables	Probability When Independent Variable Held at its Minimum	Probability When Independent Variable Held at its Maximum	Difference in Probability Max minus Min
Demographic Variables:			
Age	0.275	0.096	−0.179
Male (1 = male, 0 = female)	0.200	0.207	0.007
Black (1 = Black, 0 = White or Mixed)	0.209	0.074	−0.135
Mixed (1 = Mixed, 0 = Black or White)	0.232	0.156	−0.076
Economic Variables:			
Total personal income (logged)	0.165	0.211	0.046
Education (1 = no high school ... 17 = Doctoral Deg.)	0.092	0.312	0.220
Wealth (1 = owns home, 0 = rents home)	0.153	0.229	0.076
Occupational Prestige Index	0.195	0.217	0.022
Above Poverty Threshold (1 = 100, 5 = 500)	0.152	0.234	0.082
Acculturation Variables:			
Born in the United States (1 = yes, 0 = no)	0.134	0.302	0.168
Years in Living in the United States	0.148	0.518	0.370
English Primary Language Spoken	0.141	0.500	0.359

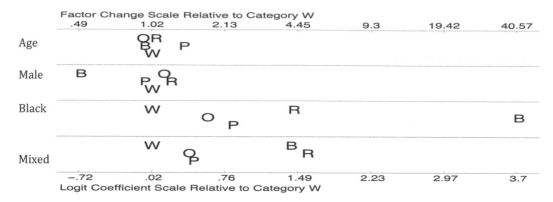

FIGURE 2   Odds of marrying different groups relative to marrying Whites by demographic variables.

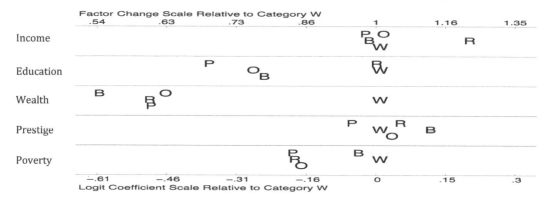

FIGURE 3   Odds of marrying different groups relative to marrying Whites by social class.

TABLE 4

HLM Multinomial Logistic Regression Predicting Marriage to Whites for Puerto Ricans in the United States (Odds Ratios)

County Level-2 Variables	Puerto Rican Married to Puerto Rican (P)	Puerto Rican Married to Other Latino (O)	Puerto Rican Married to Black (B)	Puerto Rican Married to Other Race (R)
Isolation Index (Puerto Rican/White)	10.412**	0.009**	10.794**	0.144**
Percent Puerto Rican (year 2009)	1.058**	1.063**	1.004	1.001
Social Disorganization				
Concentrated Disadvantage	0.991	1.039	1.004	0.968
Residential Instability	1.009	1.017	1.001	0.979
Ethnic Heterogeneity	4.293**	12.756**	3.068*	142.025**
Global Status Index	0.996	1.046	0.906**	0.928
Percent Low Service Occupations	0.935**	0.970	0.976	0.977
Percent Manufacturing	0.960**	1.015	0.958	0.941**
Percent Urban	0.990	1.012	1.016	0.988

Note. P = odds of a Puerto Rican marrying another Puerto Rican *relative* to *Whites*; B = Odds of a Puerto Rican marrying a Black person relative to marrying a White person, and so on. Models control for all level-1 covariates.
   $*p < .05. **p < .01.$

RESULTS

Our focus on Table 1 is on the proportion of Puerto Ricans who are married to other groups. As noted above, more than half of all Puerto Ricans (54%) are married to other Puerto Ricans, and almost a quarter (23%) are married to non-Hispanic Whites. Whereas 15% of Puerto Ricans are married to other Latinos, only 3% are married to African Americans, and even fewer (2%) are married to individuals from other backgrounds. What are the individual level characteristics that are influencing these marriage patterns?

To answer this question we turn to Table 2, which evaluates the relationship between out-marriage and demographic, economic, and acculturation variables. Here, we are primarily concerned with comparing the likelihood that Puerto Ricans marry other Puerto Ricans relative to marrying Whites (Table 2). The odds ratios can easily be interpreted in terms of percentages. For instance, for every additional year in age, Puerto Ricans have a 2% (1.023) greater chance of marrying other Puerto Ricans than having a White spouse. Note that the reference category in Table 2 is White. When compared to Puerto Rican females, Puerto Rican males are 7% (0.93) less likely to marry Puerto Ricans than to marry Whites. Put differently, Puerto Rican males are more likely to marry Whites than Puerto Rican females. Similarly, Black Puerto Ricans have a 126% (greater chance of marrying other Puerto Ricans, relative to marrying a White person, than White Puerto Ricans. That is, Black Puerto Ricans are less likely than White Puerto Ricans to marry non-Hispanic Whites. Puerto Ricans who are of mixed racial background are also less likely (152%) to marry Whites when compared to White Puerto Ricans.

Turning the focus to the effects that economic variables have on marriage patterns, still in Table 2, it appears that Puerto Ricans of greater economic means are more likely to marry non-Hispanic Whites than to marry other Puerto Ricans. Specifically, we see that as education increases, the odds of a Puerto Rican marrying another Puerto Rican, compared to marrying a White person, decrease by 14% (0.861). Among Puerto Ricans who own a home, the odds of marrying another Puerto Rican, compared to marrying a White person decrease by 50% (0.607). And among Puerto Ricans who are further away from the poverty threshold, their odds of marrying other Puerto Ricans, relative to Whites, decrease by 14% (0.869). Taken as a whole, Puerto Ricans with higher socioeconomic status (SES) are more likely to marry Whites than Puerto Ricans with lower levels of SES.

A visual representation of each marriage pattern is captured in Figures 1–3. In these multinomial odds plots, we plot the odds for each group relative to Whites. Thus, groups that appear to the right of W (for Whites) have a greater chance of marrying a particular group relative to marrying Whites. Take for instance the row for Black in Figure 1. Notice the B on the far right of the graph. This means that Black Puerto Ricans have much greater odds of marrying non-Hispanic Blacks than marrying Whites. In fact, Black Puerto Ricans have much higher odds of marrying Black African Americans than any other group. In Figure 2, we also see the effects of class. For instance, Puerto Ricans who own a home, an indicator of wealth, have a much lower likelihood of marrying any other group than marrying Whites. Notice how all the letters are to the left of the W (White) reference category. We leave the reader to explore all other marriage patterns in Figures 1–4, including the effects of acculturation variables.

Another way to make sense of these complex patterns is by looking at predicted probabilities. Specifically, we continue to focus on the probability that Puerto Ricans marry Whites. In Table 3, we present probabilities for each of the individual level variables, while holding all other variables at their respective mean. For instance, we see that Black Puerto Ricans have a .135 lower probability than White Puerto Ricans of being married to non-Hispanic Whites. Among the economic variables, education has the strongest relationship; Puerto Ricans with the highest level of education have a .220 greater probability of marrying non-Hispanic Whites than Puerto Ricans with the lowest levels of education. People who have been in the United States the longest, those

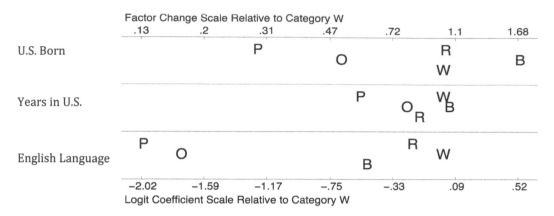

FIGURE 4 Odds of marrying different groups relative to marrying Whites by acculturation variables.

born in the United States, and those who primarily Speak English all have a greater probability of marrying Whites than their peers who have not been in the United States for very long, those who were not born in the United States, and those who speak Spanish or some other language at home, respectively.

In Table 4, we conclude our analyses by focusing on the relationship between county level-2 structural variables and inter-group marriage patterns. Again, our focus is on the likelihood that Puerto Ricans marry Whites, but we also present marriage patterns for other groups. One striking finding in Table 4 is the relationship between segregation, measured with the isolation index, and the odds of marrying Puerto Ricans relative to marrying Whites. Puerto Ricans who live in the most segregated counties (isolation = .37) are significantly more likely to marry other Puerto Ricans than to marry Whites, when compared to Puerto Ricans who live in counties where they are least segregated from Whites (isolation = 0). For instance, if we compare Puerto Ricans in the most segregated county to Puerto Ricans living in the least segregated county, then we can expect that Puerto Ricans who are most segregated from Whites have a 285% (10.412*.37) greater odds of marrying Puerto Ricans than marrying Whites, when compared to Puerto Ricans who are least segregated from Whites. This result is obtained multiplying the odds ratio coefficient in column 2 of Table 2 by the desired change in the isolation index (e.g., .37). Similarly, a ten point increase in the segregation index increases the odds that Puerto Ricans are married to Blacks by 7% (10.794*.10) when compared to marrying Whites. In fact, out of all the level-1 and level-2 variables, segregation has one of the strongest relationships with the likelihood that Puerto Ricans marry other Puerto Ricans and Blacks, relative to marrying Whites. Put differently, Puerto Ricans who live in highly segregated counties are much less likely to marry Whites than Puerto Ricans who live in less segregated counties. Segregation continues to be one of the most significant factors that impact the life chances of racial and ethnic minorities.

CONCLUSION

While few intermarriage studies have been conducted on Puerto Ricans (see Aquino, 2011), research that examines intermarriage between African Americans and Whites has contributed to a broader understanding of the possibilities and constraints of racial integration in the United States (Kincannon, 2010; Yancey, 2007). Intermarriage transforms the racial, ethnic and cultural awareness and opinions of both partners and generates offspring who may contribute to altering the views of their family members (Rosenblatt, Karis, & Powell, 1995). Because Puerto Ricans experience higher levels of intermarriage than other Latino groups, an analysis of out-marriage factors for Puerto Ricans yields important considerations for the future of Latino integration within U.S. society.

Drawing on the RPIF (Burgos & Rivera, 2012), and insights from classical and contemporary theories of assimilation, this study examined if residential segregation affects marriage patterns among Puerto Ricans living in the United States Although our focus was on whether segregation affects the likelihood of Puerto Ricans marring Whites, we also examine if segregation affects the likelihood that Puerto Ricans marry other groups (African Americans, Other Latinos, and other groups). We also explore the robustness of the segregation and intermarriage relationship by controlling for the effects of other important correlates of interracial marriages that have been identified in the literature, such as race, gender, acculturation (English language, time in the United States), and socioeconomic status (income, education, wealth, occupational prestige, and poverty). Overall, our results support the RPIF in that segregation is a significant predictor of marriage patterns, above and beyond the effects of demographic factors, and measures of acculturation and SES. Thus, residential segregation is a powerfully structural condition that shapes the incorporation of Puerto Rican migrants and their mainland born descendants in ways that call into question singularly cultural explanations.

Our findings also reveal that cultural variables like place of birth, years living in the United States and English language use were also related to likelihood that a Puerto Rican would marry a Non-Hispanic White. Puerto Ricans with greater levels of acculturation were more likely to marry Whites and less likely to marry other groups when compared to less acculturated Puerto Ricans. In addition, Puerto Ricans of higher SES were more likely to marry Whites than their lower SES peers, a finding that is consistent with classical spatial assimilation theory and segmented assimilation theory. That close to a quarter of Puerto Rican adults are married to non-Hispanic Whites indicates that a considerable segment of stateside Puerto Ricans are incorporating into mainstream U.S. society via out-marriage. These Puerto Ricans however, are Whiter, wealthier, more highly educated, and more likely to be male demonstrating a bifurcation by race, gender and socioeconomic status. These exogamous Puerto Ricans are leaving their Blacker, poorer, less educated, and female counterparts behind in highly segregated communities. Remaining in ethnic enclaves, these "left behind" Puerto Ricans are likely to be constrained within lower wage ethnic labor markets and have mixed feelings regarding the benefits of assimilation (Burton, Bonilla-Silva, Ray, Buckelew, & Hordge, 2010; Portes & Zhou, 1993; Vélez & Burgos, 2010). Puerto Ricans who marry Non-Hispanic Whites may experience stronger marriages not solely as a result of assimilation to mainstream culture but because of the stability associated with access to middle class employment markets and living in middle class communities. These Puerto Ricans are incorporating into the economic and cultural mainstream.

The finding that Puerto Rican females are less likely to marry Whites than Puerto Rican males suggests that Puerto Rican women, despite higher levels of education on average, may experience less mobility than Puerto Rican men. Although Aquino (2011) used a different statistical approach, our results contradict Aquino's findings that support Nagel's (2003) relationship between dominant group male and ethnic minority women intermarriage. On the contrary, we find that more Puerto Rican males are marrying White women more frequently Puerto Rican females marry Whites. Even as Puerto Rican women have been able to attain higher levels of educational attainment the fact that Puerto Rican males out marry Whites at a higher rate supports the original status-caste exchange theory for Puerto Ricans, although within considerably different racial and economic contexts than applied when the theory was first devised.

The finding that overall Puerto Ricans marry non-Puerto Ricans at higher rates than other Latino groups may lead to the assumption that Puerto Ricans may be more assimilated than other Latinos. However, a closer analysis takes into account crucial variables such as time in the U.S and economic and structural factors. At this moment in history ethnic incorporation patterns for some Puerto Ricans resemble the experiences of earlier European immigrants to United States, however longstanding patterns of residential segregation and economic disadvantage are not likely to abate for this community in the near future. Social workers and other mental health practitioners should not underestimate the impact of structural inequality and discrimination on the life trajectories of Puerto Ricans and other racialized minorities.

Future Research Implications

The findings of this study yield several areas for research which would further explore the dynamics of Puerto Rican/Latino intermarriage and its implications for future research. Another statistical analysis might examine the frequency of marital dissolution among intermarried Puerto Ricans as opposed to those who marry other Puerto Ricans. Higher divorce rates for intermarried couples have been documented, although research suggests that Latinos do not experience the highest divorce rates (Bratter & King, 2008). Bratter (2006) has also looked at psychological distress among interracial couples. Qualitative research would yield rich descriptions to the benefits and challenges experienced by exogamous Puerto Ricans.

Implications for Practitioners

Assimilation occurs at the crossroads of individual choices, behaviors, and structural influences. The findings of our research encourage clinicians to view Puerto Ricans with whom they work through multiple lenses as no linear model can account for all the forces that impact a particular community, family, or individual. The RPIF framework captures the complexity of institutional, cultural and interpersonal mechanisms that shape and sustain assimilation (Burgos & Rivera, 2012) and is resonant with the ecological systems and person in environment perspective (Germain & Gitterman, 1996). While Western marriage is often viewed as a deeply intimate and personal choice, it is also an indicator of assimilation and social distance (Rosenfeld, 2002). The marriage landscape of Puerto Ricans however, does not tell a uniform story of incorporation into mainstream U.S. society. In contrast, the data suggests that the gender, racial identification, socioeconomic status, and importantly the structural environment within which Puerto Ricans live will inform the type and frequency of intermarriages. Social workers and other mental health practitioners should be aware of these micro and macro forces in their work with Puerto Rican couples and families as decisions they make regarding their most intimate relationships are influenced by forces beyond their control.

Our findings also demonstrate that while exogamous Puerto Ricans may have moved "out of the barrio" and ostensibly overcome the pernicious socioeconomic effects of segregation; these moves are often accompanied by high psychosocial costs incurred by the challenges of maintaining ties with family members who remain in highly segregated Puerto Rican enclaves. For clinicians working with Puerto Ricans where intermarriage is a factor, a detailed family history should be obtained that considers these complexities. In addition, knowledge of how individual Puerto Ricans and their non-Puerto Rican spouses, and their multi-racial and multi-ethnic children understand their identity is critical in assessing family cohesion and in working to strengthen marriages and family units. These individuals and their families may be more vulnerable to acculturative stress as they navigate different racial, ethnic, linguistic and class terrain (Smart & Smart, 1995). Given the relatively high rate of intermarriage in the Puerto Rican community, the existence and nature of cultural conflict remains unmapped clinical territory.

At the micro level, the increased propensity of Puerto Ricans to intermarry with non-Hispanic Whites compared to other Latino groups will also impact the racial and ethnic identification of their offspring. At the mezzo level, raising children of mixed-race heritage in integrated communities can deeply change the racial outlook of majority group members (such as the non-Hispanic White spouses of Puerto Ricans and their extended families) by reducing inter-racial and inter-ethnic conflict which may increase their willingness to support race-specific policies like Affirmative Action (Yancey, 2007). However, the process of identity formation for these children may be impacted by tension between two or more cultures. Several empirical studies have found a relationship between high acculturation or length of time in the United States and externalizing problem behaviors such as aggression and negative peer relations in youth. They also found a relationship between ethnic identity and self-esteem, and evidence for the assertion that biculturalism is a protective factor (Smokowski, Buchanan, & Bacallao, 2009). Therefore, social work practitioners may serve their Puerto Rican and mixed race clients well by assisting them in achieving an integrated ethnic identity that positively impacts self-esteem.

While our findings emphasize the influence of structural factors, especially residential segregation which decreases the likelihood that U.S. Puerto Ricans will marry non-Hispanic Whites, many considerations remain regarding the implications of these findings. First, we do not assume that the "out of the barrio" model of assimilation will prevail in future decades as the exponential growth of the U.S. Latino population suggests an increasingly bifurcated populace, one that will be increasingly socioeconomically and residentially segregated. With this in mind, it is not probable that Puerto Ricans, who are the most likely Latinos to marry non-Hispanic Whites, will adhere to the "melting pot" model and fully incorporate into the nations' cultural and economic mainstream in the foreseeable future. Rather, if Puerto Rican out-marriage patterns are a harbinger for the U.S. Latino future; models of assimilation will be reformulated, with more than one dominant culture in regards to population yet one still subordinate in regards to economic and political power.

NOTE

1. Using this logic, it can be presumed that Blacks still have not assimilated "receptionally" through attitudes and behavior, as recent data suggests that intermarriage between Blacks, a historically stigmatized group, and Whites is still relatively lower than other groups (Rosenfeld, 2002, #568).

REFERENCES

Acevedo-Garcia, D., Lochner, K. A., Osypuk, T. L., & Subramanian, S. V. (2003). Future directions in residential segregation and health research: A multilevel approach. *American Journal of Public Health*, *93*(2), 215–221.

Acevedo-Garcia, D., & Osypuk, T. L. (2008). Impacts of housing and neighborhoods on health: Pathways, racial/ethnic disparities, and policy directions. In J. H. Carr & N. K. Kutty (Eds.), *Segregation: The rising costs for America* (pp. 197–236). New York: Routledge.

Alba, R. D., & Nee, V. (1997). Rethinking assimilation theory for a new era of immigration. *International Migration Review*, *31*(4), 826–874.

Alba, R. D., & Nee, V. (2002). *Remaking the American mainstream assimilation and contemporary immigration*. Cambridge, MA: Harvard University Press.

Aquino, G. (2011). *Puerto Rican intermarriages: The intersectionality of race, gender, class and space*. (Unpublished dissertation). State University of New York at Albany, Albany, New York.

Aranda, E. (2006). *Emotional bridges to Puerto Rico: Migration, return migration, and the struggles of incorporation*. Lanham, MD: Rowman & Littlefield.

Baird, J., Adelman, R. M., Reid, L. W., & Jaret, C. (2008). Immigrant settlement patterns: The role of metropolitan characteristics. *Sociological Inquiry*, *78*(3), 310–334.

Bell, W. (1954). A Probability model for the measurement of ecological segregation. *Social Forces*, *32*(4), 357–364.

Blau, P. M. (1977). *Inequality and heterogeneity*. New York: Free.

Blauner, B. (2001). *Still the big news: Racial oppression in America* (rev. ed.). Philadelphia, PA: Temple University Press.

Bobo, L. D., & Zubrinsky, C. L. (1996). Attitudes on residential integration: Perceived status differences, mere in-group preference, or racial prejudice. *Social Forces, 74*(3), 883–909.

Bratter, J. (2006). 'What about the couple?' Interracial marriage and psychological distress. *Social Science Research, 34*(4), 1025–1047.

Bratter, J., & King, R. B. (2008). "But will It last?": Marital instability among interracial and same-race couples. *Family Relations, 57*(2), 160–171.

Burgos, G., & Rivera, F. I. (2012). Residential segregation, socioeconomic status, and disability: A multilevel study on Puerto Ricans in the United States. *CENTRO: Journal of the Center for Puerto Rican Studies, 24*(2), 14–47.

Burton, L. M., Bonilla-Silva, E., Ray, V., Buckelew, R., & Freeman, E. H. (2010). Critical race theories, colorism, and the decade's research on families of color. *Journal of Marriage & Family, 72*(3), 440–459.

Carr, J. H., & Kutty, N. K. (2008a). *Segregation: The rising costs for America.* New York: Routledge.

Carr, J. H., & Kutty, N. K. (2008b). The new imperative for equality. In J. H. Carr & K. Kutty (Eds.), *Segregation: The rising costs for America* (pp. 1–37). New York: Routledge.

Cheong, Y. F., & Raudenbush, S. W. (2000). Measurement and structural models for children's problem behaviors. *Psychological Methods, 5*(4), 477–495.

Christensen, F. (2011). Residential segregation and Black-White intermarriage. *Economics Bulletin, 31*(2), 772–738.

Collazo, S. G., Ryan, C. L., & Bauman, K. J. (2010). *Profile of the Puerto Rican Population in United States and Puerto Rico: 2008.* Proceedings from Population Association of America, Dallas, Texas.

Davis, K. (1941). Intermarriage in caste societies. *American Anthropologist, 43,* 388–395.

De Jesús, A., & Vásquez, D. W. (2005). Exploring the Latino education profile and pipeline for Latinos in New York State. *New York Latino Research and Resources Network Policy Brief, 2.*

Duany, J. (2002). *The Puerto Rican Nation on the move: Identities on the esland & in the United States.* Chapel Hill, NC: University of North Carolina Press.

Duany, J. (2010). The Orlando Ricans: Overlapping edentity discourses among middle-class Puerto Rican immigrants. *Centro Journal, 22,* 85–115.

Duncan, O. D. (1961). A socio-economic index for all occupations. In A. J. Reiss, O. D. Duncan, P. K. Hatt, & C. C. North (Eds.), *Occupations and Social Status* (pp. 109–138). New York: Free Press.

Enchautegui, M. E., & Freeman, R. B. (2006). Why don't more Puerto Rican men work? The rich uncle (Sam) hypothesis. In S. Collins, B. Bosworth, & M. A. Soto (Eds.), *The economy of Puerto Rico: Restoring growth* (pp. 152–182). Washington, DC: Brookings Institute.

Enck-Wanzer, D. (2010). *The young lords, a reader.* New York: NYU Press.

Fu, V. K. (2007). How many melting pots? Intermarriage, panethnicity, and the Black/non-Black divide in the United States. *Journal of Comparative Family Studies, 38*(2), 215–237.

Germain, C. B., & Gitterman, A. (1996). *The life model of social work practice* (2nd ed.). New York: Columbia University Press.

Goldstein, H. (2010). *Multilevel Statistical Models (Wiley Series in Probability and Statistics)* (4th ed.). West Sussex, UK: Wiley.

Gordon, M. M. (1964). *Assimilation in American life.* New York: Oxford University Press.

Grosfoguel, R., & Georas, C. S. (2000). Coloniality of power and racial dynamics: Notes toward a reinterpretation of Latino Caribbeans in New York City. *Identities, 7*(1), 85–125.

Hosmer, D. W., & Lemeshow, S. (2000). *Applied logistic regression* (2nd. ed.). New York, NY: Wiley-Interscience Publication.

Iceland, J., & Nelson, K. A. (2010). The residential segregation of mixed-nativity married couples. *Demography, 47*(4), 869–893.

Jacobs, J. A., & Labov, T. G. (2002). Gender differentials in intermarriage among sixteen race and ethnic groups. *Sociological Forum, 17*(4), 621–646.

Kalmijn, M. (1998). Intermarriage and Homogamy: Causes, patterns, and trends. *Annual Review of Sociology, 24*(1), 395–421.

Kincannon, H. T. (2010). *Interracial marriage in the U.S. in 2006* (Unpublished doctoral dissertation). Texas A&M University, College Station, TX.

Kramer, M. R., & Hogue, C. R. (2009). Is segregation bad for your health? *Epidemiologic Reviews, 31,* 178–194.

Kubrin, C. E., & Stewart, E. A. (2006). Predicting who reoffends: The neglected role of neighborhood context in recidivism studies. *Criminology, 44*(1), 165–197.

Latkin, C., & Curry, A. (2003). Stressful neighborhoods and depression: A prospective study of the impact of neighborhood disorder. *Journal of Health and Social Behavior, 44*(1), 34–44.

Leiman, M. (2010). *The political economy of racism.* Chicago, IL: Haymarket Books.

Lichter, D. T., Carmalt, J. H., & Qian, Z. (2011). Immigration and intermarriage among Hispanics: Crossing racial and generational boundaries. *Sociological Forum, 26*(2), 241–264.

Lieberson, S. (1981). An asymmetrical approach to segregation. In C. Peach, V. Robinson, & S. J. Smith-Rex (Eds.), *Ethnic segregation in cities* (pp. 61–82). London, UK: Croom Helm.

Long, S. J. (1997). *Regression models for categorical and limited dependent variables.* Thousand Oaks, CA: Sage.

Massey, D. S., & Denton, N. A. (1993). *American apartheid: Segregation in the making of the underclass.* Cambridge, MA: Harvard University Press.

McArdle, J. J., & Hamagami, F. (1996). Multilevel models from a multiple group structural equation perspective. In G. A. Marcoulides & R. E. Schumacker (Eds.), *Advanced structural equation modeling: Issues and techniques* (pp. 89–124). Mahwah, NJ: Erlbaum.

McKee, J. B. (1993). *Sociology and the race problem: The failure of a perspective.* Urbana, IL: University of Illinois Press.

Melendez, E., & Visser, M. A. (2011). Low-wage labor, markets, and skills selectivity among Puerto Rican migrants. *Centro: Journal of the Center for Puerto Rican Studies, 23*(11), 39–63.

Merton, R. K. (1941). Intermarriage and the social structure: Fact and theory. *Psychiatry, 4,* 361–374.

Miller, F. P., Vandome, A. F., & McBrewster, J. (2009). *White flight.* Saarbrücken, Germany: Alphascript Publishing.

Muthén, B. O., & Satorra, A. (1995). Complex sample data in structural equation modeling. *Sociological Methodology, 25,* 267–316.

Muthén, L. K., & Muthén, B. O. (2010). *Mplus user's guide* (3rd. ed.). Los Angeles, CA: Muthén & Muthén.

Nagel, J. (2003). *Race, ethnicity, and sexuality: Intimate intersections, forbidden frontiers.* New York: Oxford University Press.

Oh, R. (2005). Interracial marriage in the shadows of Jim Crow: Racial segregation as a system of racial and gender subordination. *UC Davis Law Review, 39,* 1321–1352.

Osgood, D. W., & Chambers, J. M. (2000). Social disorganization outside the metropolis: An analysis of rural youth violence. *Criminology, 38*(1), 81–115.

Portes, A., & Zhou, M. (1993). The new second generation: Segmented assimilation and its variants. *The ANNALS of the American Academy of Political and Social Science, 530*(1), 74–96.

Portes, A., Fernández Kelly, P., & Haller, W. (2005). Segmented assimilation on the ground: The new second generation in early adulthood. *Ethnic and Racial Studies, 28*(6), 1000–1040.

Portes, A., & Rumbaut, R. G. (2001). *Legacies: The story of the immigrant second generation.* New York: Russell Sage Foundation.

Qian, Z., & Lichter, D. T. (2001). Measuring marital assimilation: Intermarriage among natives and immigrants. *Social Science Research, 30*(2), 289–312.

Qian, Z., & Lichter, D. T. (2007). Social boundaries and marital assimilation: Interpreting trends in racial and ethnic intermarriage. *American Sociological Review, 72*(1), 68–94.

Raudenbush, S. W., & Bryk, A. S. (2002). *Hierarchical linear models: Applications and data analysis methods.* Thousand Oaks, CA: Sage.

Reardon, S. F., Farrell, C. R., Matthews, S. A., O'Sullivan, D. O., Bischoff, K., & Firebaugh, G. (2009). Race and space in the 1990s: Changes in the geographic scale of racial residential segregation, 1990–2000. *Social Science Research, 38,* 55–70.

Roscigno, V. J., Karafin, D. L., & Tester, G. (2009). The complexities and processes of racial housing discrimination. *Social Problems, 56*(1), 49–69.

Rose, D. R. (2000). Social disorganization and parochial control: Religious institutions and their communities. *Sociological Forum, 15*(2), 339–358.

Rosenblatt, P. C., Karis, T., & Powell, R. R. (1995). *Multiracial couples: Black & white voices (Understanding Families series).* Thousand Oaks, CA: Sage.

Rosenfeld, M. J. (2002). Measures of assimilation in the marriage market: Mexican Americans 1970–1990. *Journal of Marriage & Family, 64*(1), 152–162.

Ruggles, S., Alexander, T. J., Genadek, C. A., Goeken, R., Schroeder, M. B., & Sobeck, M. (2010). Integrated Public Use Microdata Series: Version 5 [Machine-readable database]. Retrieved from http://usa.ipums.org/usa/

Rugh, J. S., & Massey, D. S. (2010). Racial segregation and the American foreclosure crisis. *American Sociological Review, 75*(5), 629–651.

Rumbaut, R. G. (1997). Assimilation and its discontents: Between rhetoric and reality. *International Migration Review, 31*(4), 923.

Sampson, R. J., & Morenoff, J. (1997). Ecological perspectives on the neighborhood context of urban poverty. In J. Brooks-Gunn, G. J. Duncan, & L. Aber (Eds.), *Neighborhood poverty, Vol II: Policy implications in studying neighborhoods* (pp. 1–22). New York: Russell Sage Foundation.

Scott, J., & Marshall, G. (Eds.). (2009). A dictionary of sociology. Retrieved from http://www.oxfordreference.com

Silver, P. (2010). 'Culture is more than Bingo and Salsa': Making Puertorriqueñidad in Central Florida. *Centro Journal, 22,* 57–83.

Smart, J. F., & Smart, D. W. (1995). Acculturative stress: The experience of the Hispanic Immigrant. *The Counseling Psychologist, 23*(1), 25–42.

Smokowski, P., Buchanan, R. L., & Bacallao, M. L. (2009). Acculturation and adjustment in Latino adolescents: How cultural risk factors and assets influence multiple domains of adolescent mental health. *The Journal of Primary Prevention, 30*(3–4), 371–393.

South, S. J., & Crowder, K. D. (1999). Neighborhood effects on family formation: Concentrated poverty and beyond. *American Sociological Review, 64*, 113–132.

Steinberg, S. (1981). *The ethnic myth: Race, ethnicity, and class in America* (1st ed.). New York: Atheneum.

Torres, A., Marzán, G., & Luecke, A. (2008). Puerto Rican outmigration from New York City: 1995–2000 (Policy Report 2.2). Retrieved from http://centropr.hunter.cuny.edu/sites/default/files/working_papers/Outmigration091108.pdf

Totti, X., & Matos Rodriguez, F. (2009). Activism and change among Puerto Ricans in New York: 1960's and 1970's. *Centro: The Journal of Puerto Rican Studies, 21*(2), 4–5.

U.S. Census Bureau. (2001a). *Census 2000 Summary File 1.* Washington, DC: Government Printing Office.

U.S. Census Bureau. (2001b). *Census 2000 Summary File 3.* Washington, DC: Government Printing Office.

U.S. Census Bureau. (2006). *Design and Methodology: American Community Survey, Technical Paper 67—Unedited Version.* Washington, DC: Government Printing Office.

U.S. Housing Scholars, & Research and Advocacy Organizations. (2008). *Residential segregation and housing discrimination in the United States: Violations of the international convention on the elimination of all forms of racial discrimination.* Washington, DC: The Poverty & Race Research Action Council and The National Fair Housing Alliance.

Vargas-Ramos, C. (2006). Settlement patterns and residential segregation of Puerto Ricans in the United States (Policy Report 1:2). Retrieved from http://centropr.hunter.cuny.edu/sites/default/files/working_papers/ACF65EF.pdf

Vélez, W., & Burgos, G. (2010). The Impact of Housing Segregation and Structural Factors on the Socioeconomic Performance of Puerto Ricans in the United States. *Centro: Journal of the Center for Puerto Rican Studies, 22*(1), 174–197.

Wilkes, R., & Iceland, J. (2004). Hypersegregation in the twenty-first century. *Demography, 41*(1), 23–36.

Williams, D. R., & Collins, C. (2001). Racial residential segregation: A fundamental cause of racial disparities in health. *Public Health Reports 116,* 404–416.

Yancey, G. (2007). *Interracial contact and social change.* Boulder, CO: Lynne Rienner Publishers.

Transnational Vietnamese American Marriages in the New Land

Peter Nguyen

School of Social Work, Virginia Commonwealth University, Richmond, Virginia, USA

This article examines the transnational marriages between Vietnamese men living abroad and Vietnamese women living in Vietnam. By presenting conceptual and cultural evidence to discern the dynamics of gender roles and marriage expectations in transnational marriages, the article seeks to uncover the uniqueness of roles and expectations within this culture. A closer look reveals possible marital issues based on incongruent expectations between the two parties, which may lead to possible mental health and domestic violence issues. Further, the article expounds on the barriers in receiving help. Practice, policy, and research suggestions are included.

The fall of Saigon officially took place in 1975 when the United States withdrew its troops, and Vietnam was replaced with a communist government. Since that time, many Vietnamese left their country to escape communism in search of economic and political freedom. Currently, there are over 2.2 million Vietnamese living abroad (Thai, 2003) and over 1.5 million Vietnamese residing in the United States (Census, 2011). This group brings with them their own traditional Eastern cultural norms such as child-rearing practices, religious traditions, collective family values, and marriage customs and patterns. In 1986, the Vietnamese government adopted a new economic policy that encourages free enterprise, free markets, and global engagement. As a result, the country has become prosperous. In 1995, Vietnam and the United States normalized their relationships, and Vietnamese living abroad, who were once prohibited from re-entry, can now return to their homeland to visit their loved ones. Vietnam's shift in economic policies has also attracted many foreign investors. The number of Vietnamese returning to visit or conduct business grew from 160,000 in 1993 to more than 1 million in the year 2000. The remittance by Vietnamese living abroad skyrocketed from $35 million in 1993 to an estimated $2 billion in 2000 (Thai, 2003). One of the by-products of this growth and access is the transnational or transpacific marriages that take place between Vietnamese living abroad and those at home. In other words, due to the ease of reentry, Vietnamese currently living in other countries can now return to their homeland to marry one of their own.

RETURNING TO MARRY

One subpopulation that has not received much attention is single Vietnamese men living overseas in Western countries who return to Vietnam to marry Vietnamese women and bring them back to their adopted country. They are the focus of this article. Specifically, I will examine the dynamics of gender roles and marriage expectations of the man and woman against the backdrop of the traditional Vietnamese culture versus the evolving modern culture of Vietnam. On the surface, these transnational marriages may appear to be headed for a seamless transition since there may be cultural similarities between the two parties. However, a closer examination of the literature reveals that the economic growth in Vietnam and time abroad may have contributed to ideological shifts in marital relationships and expectations between men aboard and women in Vietnam.

It should be noted that an extensive literature review did not find empirical studies that examine this specific Vietnamese subpopulation and issues involved in transnational marriages. As such, this article attempts to build on what is available in the descriptive and conceptual literature indicating the change in Vietnam and its impact on family and relationship dynamics. Moreover, it is not my intent to say that all Vietnamese couples involved in transnational marriages face these issues but, rather, to focus on possible trials and tribulations that some couples may face given the cultural shift.

Currently the number of Vietnamese returning to Vietnam to marry is not known although existing literature seems to indicate that more men return home to marry than women (Goodkind, 1997; Thai, 2003). Several hypotheses have been proposed to explain this phenomenon. Goodkind (1997) refers to the "double marriage squeeze" where there was a high male mortality rate during the Vietnam War and a large number of men emigrating to foreign countries. Thus, there has been a high ratio of males to females living abroad and vice versa and a low ratio of males to females living in Vietnam. Thai argues that in addition to the uneven immigration pattern, "Vietnamese women living overseas are much more likely than men to marry outside their ethnic group" (p. 57). Facilitation of transnational marriages can take place by reliance on the transnational family networks that will arrange the marriage or the Vietnamese press carried advertisements from men seeking brides from Vietnam.

FAMILY TRADITIONS, VALUES, AND EXPECTATIONS

The traditional Vietnamese culture is greatly influenced by the teaching of the philosopher Confucius who was born in China during the Chou Dynasty. His teaching spread when north Vietnam was annexed and ruled by China for many years. Confucius's teaching emphasizes a hierarchical family structure, in which persons at the top of the hierarchy make decisions relevant to those below them (Nguyen & Williams, 1988). More specifically, the family structure has a clearly defined hierarchy, which puts the father or husband at the pinnacle of authority and responsibility (Webb, 2001). Women have traditionally held lower status and possessed less power than men. The ideal woman is expected to submit to her father before marriage, to submit to her husband during marriage, and to submit to her adult son after her husband's death. Her principal responsibilities are to rear the children, manage the household, maintain family harmony, and sacrifice herself for her husband and children (Bowman & Edwards, 1984). Furthermore, the teaching of Confucius emphasizes family piety where children are expected to live with their biological family until they are married and show gratitude by continuing to care for their parents as they age. The father's words are dogmatic, and his authority on the children is unquestioned. This type of authoritarian parenting style is very common in the Asian culture (Arrindell et al., 1994; Best, Hose, Barnard, & Spicker, 1994; Papps, Walker, Trimboli, & Trimboli, 1995). For women, they are expected to move into the home of the husband and also help provide care for their parents-in-law. Thus, in some cases, it is the woman's responsibility to help provide care for her own parents as well as the parents of her husband. In short, the cultural prescription for the woman is based on her roles of preserving the family while autonomy and personal freedom are deemed not as important or secondary. As a result of these values, the teaching of Confucianism continues to be "a great challenge to the struggle for the equity and equal rights of Vietnamese women" (Phan, 2008, p. 178).

On the other hand, the husband assumes the role of leadership and authority and is the provider and protector of the family (Lee, 1997). He is expected to be active, aggressive, and dominating. As a leader of the family, he "will not allow his wife to make decisions without his consent ... whether his wife accepts them or not" (Phan, 2008, p. 181). Interestingly, Phan also points out that culturally men have the right to teach their wives to behave properly, and even violence is then accepted as a cultural norm by women who have learned to accept his behavior as part of their fate.

SHIFTING NORMS FOR VIETNAMESE WOMEN

The modernization of Vietnam has produced positive economic impacts on its citizens and the infrastructure of the country. However, this has also contributed to the delay of marriage for some Vietnamese women. For example, Vietnam's economic growth and entry into global markets have given women in Vietnam more opportunities in education and employment; thus making them less dependent on men as providers. This hinders some marriages since culturally Vietnamese men do not want their wives to be better than they, especially in regard to educational level or income. It is believed that "women who pursue higher education and professional careers violate the traditional role of the subservient female" (Suh, 2007, p. 31).

On the other hand, the families of well-to-do or educated women also are raising their standards in choosing a mate for their daughters. This economic shift also challenges the teaching of Confucius as women seek more of an egalitarian relationship rather than subscribing to the traditional paternalistic roles described earlier. Thai (2003) found that up to 70% of the transpacific brides who have college degrees believe that men in Vietnam do not treat women equally. Instead of being submissive and passive, they believe that they should have more involvement and input into the relationship and decision-making process. Further, the shortage of men in Vietnam due to past wars and emigration and this shift in gender role expectations have allowed Vietnamese women to be more selective when it comes to choosing their mates. This is further exacerbated when women in Vietnam have the perception that Vietnamese men living overseas are more modern and much more likely to embrace gender equality. For example, by marrying men overseas they believe that they will be in a nuclear family rather than moving in and caring for the extended family or in-laws. Or they assume that Vietnamese men are not as dominant, welcome their input in the relationship, and are open to sharing house duties. Thai (2003) asserts that this perception comes "from a variety of sources, such as films that depict overseas men as egalitarian, caring, and 'loving' to women" (p. 60) and also from relatives overseas. Last, some women can also afford to wait and be selective given their self-sufficient independence or, for some, they can wait given the help of remittance from relatives living abroad. In essence, there is a difference in gender role expectations between the Vietnamese men abroad and women in Vietnam. Durkheim's theory of social integration/regulation may help increase the understanding of this phenomenon. He stated that "rapid social change (industrialization and urbanization) creates a collective state of ambivalence; older traditional values become blurred and a new set of values are variably accepted." (Yip et al., 2012). In this context, the economic boom in Vietnam plays a role in evolution of the traditional Confucius values in modern Vietnamese society and challenges the traditional expectations of Vietnamese men who live abroad.

EXPECTATIONS OF VIETNAMESE MEN ABROAD

Thai (2003) found in his study that Vietnamese men living overseas "emphasized the need for respect" (p. 63) when it came to marriage. He found that some Vietnamese men living in the United States perceived that Vietnamese women in the United States "don't share the same Vietnamese values" (p. 64) as they do. Indeed, scholars have found that immigrant women often challenged traditional gender relations in the household and family after migration (Thai). On the contrary, Thai found that some Vietnamese men living overseas continued to have some traditional role expectations of women and expressed concerns that the woman in the United States may be materialistic, too independent, and would not provide the same level and type of care as traditionally expected. As a result, the Vietnamese men "here" presumed that they may be better matched with Vietnamese women living in Vietnam "there" since they may have preserved traditional Confucius ideologies and were better suited in terms of marital beliefs. This thinking is enforced by the gender roles as espoused by Confucius where the men and boys are highly valued and women and girls are expected to serve more submissive roles. Consequently, any challenges from the woman or wife are considered disrespectful and offend the husband's manhood. Further, he may also appear "weak" to the people in his community.

Courtship and Marriage

Today's world has shrunk, and human relationships can be easier to develop given the ease of travel and the advances in communication such as Skype, Facebook, e-mail, online dating services, and a host of other technologies. However, the limited time spent during the transnational courtship or communication via technology can obscure the relationship dynamics of everyday life and interaction of a couple. The subpopulation of Vietnamese men and women involved in transnational marriages may face difficulties in their marriage upon arriving in the United States, given the almost diametrical presumptions of values, culture, and gender roles and expectations from one another. In other words, the beginning of the marriage and the initial adjustments can be difficult for couples, but these Vietnamese couples must also deal with the challenge of reconciling the different presumptions and expectations of one another.

For Vietnamese women who come to the United States expecting an egalitarian relationship, hoping for opportunities in the United States to better themselves, and wanting to help family members back home, they must now deal with disappointments and fear. Some may be socially isolated if they have no support system such as friends or other family members. Compounding the lack of support, some of the woman also face the stressors of acculturation as they adjust from the "collectivist" way of life in Vietnam to the more dominant "individualistic" values of the U.S. society. Additionally, it can be disorienting as they learn to navigate the web of U.S. institutions and daily living in Western society. Those who do not speak English and have no mode of transportation to travel to seek employment become much more dependent on their husbands for everyday survival. Moreover, difficulties faced by the women are exacerbated when she is expected by the husband and his family to carry out the traditional duties of a wife. Brown, Hook, and Glick (2008) state that "research on marriage and gender roles suggests that 'traditional' familial norms are reinforced among newly-arrived immigrants, particularly in times of hardship" (p. 533).

Divorce is the last option should the relationship run its course; however, Vietnamese culture highly discourages divorce for it is uncommon in Vietnam. This may be due to the fact that many Vietnamese are Catholic. Further, according to Confucius's teaching, marriages help stabilize society and, therefore, divorces can serve as a destabilizing force. Thus, divorce is considered a taboo in Vietnamese society that carries a stigma and shame. Another factor that discourages divorce is the cultural value that divorced women are viewed as "damaged" since virginity and purity of the woman is valued (Phan, 2008). This is based on the belief that "an intact hymen at marriage is perceived to entail happy families, healthy children and unworried parents" (Rydstrom, 2006, p. 288). Thus, a divorced woman may be shunned by the community and discouraged against prospects of future relationships. In summary, conflicts arise due to different gender role expectations between the man and the woman but often go unresolved since the relationship is dictated by her husband. This helps reinforce the traditional gender roles. Further, this also creates dependency for the woman since she would have limited knowledge and access to resources in the community.

Mental Health Risks

Currently, there are no empirical studies examining the divorce rate, suicide rate, prevalence of domestic violence, and mental health issues for this particular subpopulation. However, it is reasonable to assume that such strained relationships can impact mental health and even contribute to domestic violence. Kanukollu and Mahalingam (2011) found that there is a higher level of acculturative stress and greater difficulty in psychological functioning when there is a greater difference between the natal and new culture. However, Asians and especially those less acculturated (Kanukollu & Mahalingam) are not likely to seek therapy due to structural and cultural barriers. Specifically,

> structural barriers (e.g., high costs, transportation inaccessibility of services, language, lack of indige-nous workers) are factors relating to one's socioeconomic or immigrant status whereas cultural barriers (e.g., shame, stigma, discrimination, perception that psychological illness as somatic, privacy) involve conflicts between one's cultural belief system and aspects of Western mental health care. (Wong et al., 2006, p. 1116)

Further, Asian women are unlikely to seek help from services in the mainstream society such as hospitals, shelters, or lawyers (Bui & Morash, 2007) since some women also do not want to be "viewed as 'mentally weak' and as inadequate wives and mothers" (Singh & Hays, 2008, p. 98). Researchers have repeatedly documented that this population either rarely uses or certainly underutilizes available mental health services (Uba, 1982); and tends to show longer delay for treatment compared to African Americans and Caucasians (Shin, 2002). Finally, they are more likely to terminate treatment prematurely in comparison to other ethnic groups (Li & Browne, 2000). This is alarming given the increase in the Asian population. To date, there have been few improvements in addressing the mental health needs of this community. Cultural factors continue to persist while external factors such as specific policies focusing on educating the Asian community about mental health are void. Further, there is a lack of bilingual or Asian mental health professionals available to work with this population.

The Potential for Domestic Violence

Due to the strains in the relationship mentioned above, it is possible that domestic violence could take place since "men who hold traditional beliefs about the male gender role are at risk to experience a great deal of stress in situations where this role is challenged" (Gallaher & Parrott, 2011, p. 570). In other words, stress experienced by the Vietnamese men in this case may be a factor in triggering domestic violence. The women may remain silent and not report to authorities because of Confucian teaching and Vietnamese society expectations that "women should silently cope with violence" (Phan, 2008, p. S178). In other cases, women may not reach out for help because they fear their husband, do not want to undermine his authority, want to hide the problem, and adhere to the overall emphasis of preserving the harmony in the family or for their children. Again, the importance of values of "privacy" and "face" can be powerful and overriding factors that dictate the women's help-seeking behavior. Another factor that contributes to the lack of seeking help is that "consistent with Vietnamese traditions, some women believe they had to endure abuse because it was their fate or the consequence of their bad deeds in previous lives" (Bui & Morash, p. 383). Thus, instead of going to seek help, these women believe that they must accept their "fate."

The barriers that prevent seeking help when domestic violence occurs is of great concern for this population in which there is a strong emphasis on paternalistic values. Yllo (1983, 1984 as cited in Bhanot & Senn, 2007, p. 26) found "positive correlations between the presence of more patriarchal social structures and higher rates of violence against women" while Bhanot and Senn (2007) found "strong empirical support for the connection between traditional gender role attitudes and attitudes that support violence against women" (p. 26). Further, research by Bui and Morash (1999) found that there is a significant positive correlation of physical abuse by a husband and a husband's traditional gender role attitudes in the Asian community. And, according to Kim and Sung (2000), the rates of wife beating are four times higher in male-dominant couples relative to egalitarian couples. Again, there are no statistics that specifically focus on this particular subpopulation and the circumstances involved.

RECOMMENDATIONS FOR PRACTICE

The Vietnam economy continues to thrive, and its economic relationship with the United States remains vibrant. It can be assumed that transnational marriages will continue to take place given the harmonious relationship of the two countries and the ease of travel. Thai (2003) asserted that marriage is the number-one reason why people migrate to the United States Therefore, it is important to find ways that can address issues that arise from these transnational marriages.

Raising Awareness

The Vietnamese community in the United States has grown large enough where native media such as television, radio, and Internet, newspapers, and magazines have populated to meet the demands. These resources are also accessible to Vietnamese people back home. Such media resources can provide education on a mass level about evolving gender roles, communication effectiveness, negotiation and conflict resolutions, and issues regarding mental health and domestic violence.

Using Cultural Values as Tools

Asking couples already living in the United States to attend "couples therapy" may not be the solution since therapy is not the most popular form of intervention in Vietnam. Therapy is viewed as focusing on "disease" or "people with problems." This is not unusual given the focus on "face" and "status" in the community. Therefore, reframing an intervention as "education" with the focus on harmony may be more apt since harmony is the main focus in the teachings of Confucius. This would be especially effective if children are involved since "Asians focus more on the parent-child relationship than the couples' relationship" (Huang, 2005, p. 169). Put differently, by explaining that the health and happiness of the child are dependent on the harmony of the home and its relationships, Vietnamese parents are more apt to receive help since the well-being of the child is at the forefront.

Using Peer Influence

Bhanot and Senn (2007) suggest "that peers can have an influence on people's conceptions of gender roles" (p. 30). They found that South Asian men who interact with non-Asian men tend to reevaluate and change their beliefs about gender roles and become more egalitarian. Although this interaction cannot be assumed or enforced, perhaps Vietnamese men who may be open to learning and self-growth can make a conscious effort for possible change by interaction with other men whom they encounter.

Identify "Brokers" and Linking to External Networks

Vietnamese women who are exposed to relationship troubles or dealing with domestic violence may not want to disclose the people in their immediate networks (family, family friends, social services, or religious institution within the community) due to fear of shame, embarrassment, or lack of confidentiality. Therefore it is important to form "brokers" in the community who can confidently serve as educators and use sound judgment to link the women to the external network (police, lawyers, government institutions).

RECOMMENDATIONS FOR POLICY

In addition to practice recommendations, policies need to be implemented in order to effectively address issues face by this population. It is worth noting that though the issue of transnational marriage of Vietnamese population is the focus of this article, more attention needs to be dedicated to the mental health of Asian Americans.

Utilizing "Insiders"

A search of the literature review regarding transnational marriages reveals very few studies in particular for the Vietnamese population. This may be due to the cultural barriers that prevent many researchers from gaining entry. Vietnamese culture values privacy, as the family's "dirty laundry" is kept quiet, and families tend to present a harmonious front. However, like other immigrant populations, Vietnamese immigrants are not immune to issues impacting their families and communities. Due to its closed system of not allowing "outsiders" to enter, there is a need to have policies that provide incentives to gain entry. One approach is by recruiting and train Vietnamese living in the community or "insiders." In this capacity, family issues involving marriage or domestic violence can best be addressed with those who are familiar with the culture and speak the same language. Further, this approach can also build capacity to research issues impacting this population and devise preventative measures.

Recruiting Mental Health Professionals

Utilizing "insiders" may be an effective way to work with the Vietnamese community from within. However, these "insiders" may lack the expertise to deal with issues that require clinical skills. In other words, there needs to be recruitment of Asians to obtain college degree pertaining to the mental health professions. The Asian population is one of the fastest-growing populations in the United States and, yet, anecdotal evidence indicates that the number of Asian mental health professionals is lacking. As such, recruitment of Asians to enter the mental health profession is of utmost importance in order to keep up with the Asian population's growth and issues that may arise.

Funding Research

Evidence-based practice has been the trend of social work practice and other mental health professions. Though there have been suggestions of interventions in working with Asian Americans, there are few research exploring its efficacy and effectiveness. One area that requires particular attention is the funding for longitudinal studies involving intervention with the Asian population and Vietnamese in particular.

RECOMMENDATIONS FOR FUTURE RESEARCH

It is important to note that there is no extensive empirical research done for Vietnamese couples who are married under transnational circumstances. This article provides a starting point on which to build future research based on conceptual and cultural evidence. It by no means assumes that every transnationally married Vietnamese couple faces the issues of incongruence of gender role expectations and value differences and must deal with mental health issues and domestic violence. Due to the lack in empirical evidence, it does offer future research questions such as examining the views of this population regarding the gender roles and impact of Confucian teaching and modern society expectations. Further, inquiries regarding communication patterns, conflict resolutions, and ways of attaining help are important to explore.

REFERENCES

Arrindell, W. A., Perris, C., Eisemann, M., Van derEnde, J., Gasner, P., Iwaawki, S., ... Zhang, J. (1994). Parental-rearing behavior from a cross-cultural perspective: A summary of data obtained in 14 nations. In C. Perris, W. A. Arrindell, & M. Eisemann (Eds.), *Parenting and psycholopathology* (pp. 145–171). New York, NY: John Wiley.

Best, D. L., House, A. S., Barnard, A. E., & Spicker, B. S. (1994). Parent-child interactions in France, Germany, and Italy: The effects of gender and culture. *Journal of Cross-Cultural Psychology, 25*, 181–193.

Bhanot, S., & Senn, C. Y. (2007). Attitudes towards violence against women in men of south Asian ancestry: Are acculturation and gender role attitudes important factors? *Journal of Family Violence, 22*, 25–31.

Bowman, B., & Edwards, M. (1984). The Indochinese refugee: An overview. *Australian and New Zealand Journal of Psychiatry, 18*, 40–52.

Brown, S. L., Van Hook, J., & Glick, J. E. (2008). Generational differences in cohabitation and marriage in the U.S. *Population Research and Policy Review, 27*, 531–550.

Bui, H. N., & Morash, M. (2007). Social capital, human capital, and reaching out for help with domestic violence: A case study of women in a Vietnamese-American community. *Criminal Justice Studies, 20*(4), 375–390.

Gallagher, K. E., & Parrott, D. J. (2011). What accounts for men's hostile attitudes toward women? The influence of hegemonic male role norms and masculine gender role stress. *Violence Against Women, 17*(5), 568–583.

Goodkind, D. (Spring, 1997). The Vietnamese double marriage squeeze. *International Migration Review, 31*(1), 108–127.

Huang, W. J. (2005). An Asia perspective on relationship and marriage education. *Family Process, 44*(2), 161–173.

Kanukollu, S. N., & Mahalingam, R. (2011). The idealized cultural identities model on help-seeking and child sexual abuse: A conceptual model for contextualizing perceptions and experiences of south Asian Americans. *Journal of Child Sexual Abuse, 20*, 218–243.

Kim, J. Y., & Sung, K. (2000). Conjugal violence in Korean American families: A residue of the cultural tradition. *Journal of Family Violence, 15*(4), 331–345.

Lee, E. (Ed.). (1997). Overview: The assessment and treatment of Asian American families. In E. Lee (Ed.), *Working with Asian American: A guide for clinicians* (pp. 3–36). New York, NY: The Guilford Press.

Li, H. Z., & Browne, A. J. (2000). Defining mental health illness and accessing mental health services: Perspectives of Asian Canadians. *Canadian Journal of Community Mental Health, 19*, 143–159.

Nguyen, N. A., & Williams, H. L. (1988). Transition from East to West: Vietnamese adolescents and their parents. *Journal of the American Academy of Child Adolescent Psychiatry, 28*, 505–515.

Papps, F., Walker, M., Trimboli, A., & Trimboli, C. (1995). Parental discipline in Anglo, Greek, Lebanese, and Vietnamese cultures. *Journal of Cross-Cultural Psychology, 26*, 49–64.

Phan, T. T. H. (2008). Sexual coercion within marriage in Quang Tri, Vietnam. *Culture, Health & Sexuality*, S177–S187.

Rydstrom, H. (2006). Sexual desires and 'social evils': Young women in rural Vietnam. *Gender, Place and Culture, 13*(3), 283–301.

Shin, J. K. 2002. Help-seeking behaviors by Korean immigrants for depression. *Issues in Mental Health Nursing, 23*(5), 461–476.

Singh, A. A., & Hays, D. G. (2008). Feminist group counseling with south Asian women who have survived intimate partner violence. *The Journal for Specialists in Group Work, 33*(1), 84–102.

Suh, S. H. (2007, Autumn). Asian women past and present: A closer look at the meaning of tradition. *Encounter, 20*(3), 31–33.

Thai, H. C. (2003). The Vietnamese double gender revolt: Globalizing marriage options in the twenty-first century. *Amerasia Journal, 29*(1), 51–74.

Uba, L. (1982). Meeting the mental health needs of Asian Americans: Mainstream or segregated services. *Professional Psychology: Research & Practice, 13*(2), 215–221.

U.S. Bureau of the Census. (2011). The Asian population in the United States. Retrieved from http://www.census.gov/population/www.census.gov/population/www.socdemo/race/Asian-US.pdf

Webb, N. B. (2001). *Culturally diverse parent-child and family relationships: A guide for social workers and other practitioners.* New York, NY: Columbia University Press.

Wong, C. E., Marshall, G. N., Schell, T. L., Elliot, M. N., Hambarsoomians, K., Chun, C. A., ... Berthold, M. S. (2006). Barriers to mental health care utilization for U.S. Cambodian refugees. *Journal of Consulting and Clinical Psychology, 74*(6), 1116 1120.

Yip, P. S. F., Ying, Y. C., Yousuf, S., Lee, K. M. C., Kawano, K., Routley, V., ... Wu, K. C. C. (2012). Towards a reassessment of the role divorce in suicide outcomes: Evidence from five pacific rim populations. *Social Science & Medicine, 75*, 358–366.

"First Train Out": Marriage and Cohabitation in the Context of Poverty, Deprivation, and Trauma

Naomi Farber

College of Social Work, University of South Carolina, Columbia, South Carolina, USA

Julie E. Miller-Cribbs

Anne and Henry Zarrow School of Social Work, University of Oklahoma-Tulsa, Tulsa, Oklahoma, USA

There has been a steep rise in the proportion of children born to and living with unmarried parents. Unmarried parents are increasingly likely to cohabitate, especially low-income couples, placing their children at elevated psychosocial risk. This life history study of poor, White single mothers suggests that the current focus on differences between married and cohabiting poor women may overstate underlying similarities in factors associated with their partner formation and dissolution and that poor women's decisions about marriage and cohabitation must be understood in a developmental context that reflects the stacking, over time, of multiple forms of vulnerability to unstable partnerships, single motherhood, and continuing poverty into adulthood.

INTRODUCTION

Over the past several decades, there have been important changes in patterns of family formation in the United States contributing to the steep rise in the proportion of children born to and living with unmarried parents. Although it is not clear yet whether or not these shifts represent genuine alterations in norms regarding the basic structural context of family formation, there is widespread concern over growing instability in contemporary family life (Raley & Bumpass, 2003). While these changes are occurring broadly throughout American society, low-income men and women are considerably more likely to have and to raise children outside of marriage and thus to place themselves and their children at risk for numerous forms of disadvantage.

In response to these changes, the recent public policies intended to encourage marriage and to discourage childbearing outside of marriage focus particularly on low-income families as a strategy to reduce poverty and welfare costs (Lichter, Graefe, & Brown, 2003). Underlying this formal effort to influence individuals' decisions about family formation is an assumption that marriage carries important symbolic meaning and practical advantages to parents and their children. Despite evidence that marriage is associated with more positive lifelong outcomes than

This work was funded in part by the Lois and Samuel Silberman Fund, New York Community Trust.

cohabitation or single parenthood for adults and children, for severely disadvantaged women marriage may not necessarily confer such benefits. We add to this discourse in comparing the experiences of formation and dissolution of marital and cohabiting unions among White low-income single mothers in a non-metro Southern context. Drawing on life history data, we contend: first, that the current focus on the differences between married and cohabiting poor women may overstate significant underlying similarities in factors associated with their partner formation and dissolution; and second, that poor women's decisions about marriage and cohabitation must be understood in a developmental context that reflects the convergence, or stacking, over time, of multiple forms of vulnerability to unstable partnerships, single motherhood, and continuing poverty into adulthood.

BACKGROUND

Despite consistent evidence that Americans continue to value marriage as a cultural ideal and personal aspiration, the structural contours of family formation in the United States have changed significantly over the last several decades (Gibson-Davis, Edin, & McLanahan, 2005). The convergence of these changes is starkly evident in the significant decrease in the proportion of children who grow up in families that include their married biological parents. This results in part from the intersection of several demographic transformations over many decades, including the decline in marriage and marital fertility, increase in the average age at marriage, increase in divorce, and decrease in remarriage (Brown, Sanchez, Nock, & Wright, 2006; Ellwood & Jencks, 2006; Goldstein & Kenney, 2001). Among the most striking of recent developments is the steady and substantial increase in children who are born to unmarried mothers, rising from 3.8% in 1940 to 38.5% of all American children in 2006 (Solomon-Fears, 2008). The likelihood of bearing a child outside of marriage is especially high for low-income women. About a third of poor women over age 25 have had a child outside of marriage in contrast to only 5% of more affluent women (Edin, 2000). In sharp contrast to the past, when nonmarital pregnancy often resulted in a "shotgun" marriage, fewer single women who become pregnant today marry the fathers of their children (Seltzer, 2000).

While unmarried pregnant women are less likely now to marry, single mother families increasingly include cohabiting parents. Currently, about half of unmarried mothers are cohabiting with their child's father (Waldfogel, Craigie, & Brooks-Gunn, 2010). Cohabitation is more likely to occur among minority and poor couples, and those with lower levels of education (Blackwell & Lichter, 2000; Bumpass & Lu, 2000; Lichter, Qian, & Mellott, 2006; Lichter & Qian, 2008; Manning & Smock, 2005; Smock, 2000; Teitler & Reichman, 2001). However, the magnitude of this change is especially notable among Whites, among whom increases in non-marital childbearing "... appear to have been driven almost entirely by increases in births within cohabiting unions ..." (Wu, Bumpass, & Musick, 2001, p. 4). While cohabitation among more affluent couples often serves as a trial period leading to marriage, unions among poor cohabiting couples tend to be less stable. Poor couples' cohabiting relationships are of shorter duration and are more likely to end in dissolution, with only a third marrying within 5 years (Bumpass & Lu, 2000; Lichter et al., 2006; Smock, Manning, & Porter, 2005). Although pregnancy and childbearing increase the likelihood that cohabitation will result in marriage, it is a less likely outcome among poor women who do not have a high school diploma (Harknett & McLanahan, 2004; Smock, 2000; Edin, 2000; Smock et al., 2005; Seltzer, 2000).

Among the reasons for concern about nonmarital childbearing and child rearing is the mounting evidence that growing up in a single-parent family poses significant risks to children's well-being across the lifespan, including reduced educational attainment, behavioral and emotional problems, poor health, early sexual activity and pregnancy, and later poverty (Currie & Stabile, 2006;

Moore, Redd, Burkhauser, Mbwana, & Collins, 2009; Solomon-Fears, 2008). Recent research finds that marriage between biological parents provides the most advantageous of all family contexts for children's development. In comparison to living with married parents, children in cohabiting families are more likely to be poor—8.5% and 42.9%, respectively; to experience transitions in family structure; and to be physically and/or sexually abused; (DeKlyen, Brooks-Gunn, McLanahan, & Knab, 2006; Seltzer, 2000; Smock, 2000; Moore et al., 2009; Waldfogel et al., 2010; Whelan, 1994). There is no consensus regarding the reasons for this overall benefit, but it appears that the greater stability associated with marriage is one critical factor in positive child outcomes.

Despite the apparent advantages of marriage in general, the prevailing scholarly focus on distinctions between romantic couples who choose marriage versus cohabitation may not capture sufficiently the complex and variable lifelong patterns of partnership found among poor women with children. Among women born since 1945, approximately 20% of nonmarital births occurred within a cohabitating union that formed after the dissolution of a first marriage (Brown et al., 2006). After the dissolution of a marriage, White women are more likely than African American and Hispanic women to give birth while unmarried (Wu, 2008). The sequence of childbearing and types of partnership may influence subsequent choices, as women who have children outside of marriage dramatically decrease their chances of later marrying; and, if they marry, they tend to marry men who possess characteristics that make them less attractive marital partners (Lichter & Graefe, 2007; Lichter & Qian, 2008).

In reviewing recent research about barriers to marriage among poor women and men, Edin and Reed (2005) suggest that both social and economic factors play a role in their marital decisions. They find that while disadvantaged women and men value marriage and expect to marry in the future, they do not assume that that "childbearing and marriage as life events go together" (p. 128). Given this belief, held in the context of high expectations for economic stability for a successful marriage and low earnings of men, antipathy toward divorce, relationship quality, the likelihood of bringing to the union children from other partners, marriage may carry more risk than promise. These reasons thus support, in essence, a multidimensional version of the predominant perspective assuming that decisions about marriage represent at least partially rational choices about family formation (Becker, 1981). While all of these barriers are composed of multiple elements that interact in complex ways, those characteristics and experiences that define relationship quality are particularly complicated and less easily understood as expressions of rational calculations. In addition to the many relevant substantive factors, there are temporal dimensions that must be considered if we are to understand their mechanisms of influence on partnership choice among poor women who have children.

RELATIONSHIP QUALITY, UNION FORMATION, AND DISSOLUTION

There is consistent evidence that relationship quality is a primary factor in poor women's decisions about forming as well as dissolving both marital and cohabiting unions with men (Cherlin et al., 2004; Lichter et al., 2006). Several factors identified by poor women as deterrents from marrying also occur in cohabitating relationships, including physical and emotional abuse, substance abuse, and infidelity. Often these problems coexist and serve as the impetus for termination of the relationship (Reed, 2007; Edin & Kefalas, 2005). Poor women are more susceptible to being victims of domestic violence, particularly White women (Edin & Kefalas, 2005; Farber & Miller-Cribbs, in press; Jasinski, 2004). Edin (2000) finds that for poor White women, lack of trust and domestic violence are especially significant influences on in their partnership histories.

Recent research suggests that the impact of stress on dyadic adult relationships is a growing, though insufficiently understood problem (Randall & Bodenmann, 2009). Poor couples experiencing material hardship are especially vulnerable to the negative impact of life stressors or "hassles" found to be associated with marital satisfaction and functioning (Cohan & Bradbury, 1997; Crnic & Avevdo, 1995). The cumulative stress can deplete the capacity to cope effectively with the demands of parenting and partner relationships, sometimes because of poor problem solving capacities (Cohan & Bradbury, 1997; Webster-Stratton, 1990).

Some poor individuals enter unions with heightened vulnerability to the impact of these stresses as a result of preexisting characteristics such as mental illness (Teitler & Reichman, 2008) as well as early experiences that may compromise healthy development. There is increasing focus on the impact of childhood trauma, particularly physical or sexual abuse on relationship quality in adulthood, including marital disruption and satisfaction (Cohan & Bradbury, 1997; Cherlin et al., 2004; Fergusson, Horwood, & Lynskey, 1997; Whisman, 2006; Liang, Williams, & Siegel, 2006; Nelson & Wampler, 2000). The experience of violence in childhood is associated with later problems with intimacy, trust, sexual relations, and emotional and physical well-being (Briere, 1992; Edward et al., 1999). The potential effects of maltreatment, such as posttraumatic stress disorder (PTSD), can influence relationships across the lifespan, particularly evident when a maltreated child attempts to form a new relationship with a primary caregiver or later romantic or marital partner (Cicchetti & Blender, 2004). For example, symptoms of PTSD such as flashbacks, irritability, hyperarousal, sexual problems, and detachment can create barriers to forming and maintaining healthy and stable relationships through increasing communication problems and reducing intimacy between partners (Davis & Petretic-Jackson, 2000; Whisman, 2006). Sexual abuse, in particular, may especially threaten the capacity for sustainable adult relationships in its effect on both male and female victims' capacity for intimacy and healthy sexuality (Finkelhor, Hotaling, Lewis, & Smith, 1989; DiLillo, 2001; Rumstein-McKean & Hunsley, 2001; Cherlin et al., 2004; Kia-Keating, Sorsoli, & Grossman, 2009). Experiencing multiple forms of traumas may contribute to suffering even greater relationship difficulties as adults (Cloitre, Tardiff, Marzuk, Leon, & Portera, 1996; Wind & Silvern, 1992). Women who experience trauma as children also are at elevated risk for adult victimization through rape, interpersonal violence, dating violence, and having multiple sexual partners (Ararata, 2000; Gidycz, Hanson, & Layman, 1995; Boney-McCoy & Finkelhor, 1996; Fergusson et al., 1997; Himelein, 1995). Arata and Lindman (2002) propose that women who leave home early to escape sexual abuse and then marry at a young age may be at higher risk for further re-victimization. They suggest that, "Rather than early marriage serving as a mediating variable, it is possible that the types of abuse that are associated with a desire to leave the home early may also be the types that increase risk for re-victimization" (Arata & Lindman, 2002, p. 966).

Thus, there is growing evidence that the consequences of childhood trauma such as being a victim, as well as a witness of domestic abuse may be experienced across the lifespan into adult relationships. This study addresses the need for more nuanced understanding of both intrapersonal and interpersonal processes that affect decisions about cohabitation and marriage through examining the salience of childhood trauma and other forms of vulnerability for particular decisions about partnerships and family formation among poor, White single mothers.

CURRENT STUDY

This study was conceived to explore broadly reasons for the comparatively high incidence of nonmarital childbearing among White and African American single mothers in the context of Southern rural poverty using a life history method. A forthcoming report on these data focuses on the salience of stacked vulnerabilities, especially exposure to childhood and early adult violence, for the formation of social capital among poor White single mothers. Here we expand this lifespan analysis of stacked vulnerabilities in examining the women's perceived motivations for their specific decisions about marriage and cohabitation with the fathers of their children and in other central romantic relationships. While existing research affirms the significance of partner choice in the trajectories of both marital and cohabiting unions, there has been less attention paid to the reasons that poor women may choose these partners beyond accounting for the limits of the available pool of men and theories of mate selection (Wilson, 1987; Edin & Reed, 2005). We contribute to this line of research through examining the circumstances surrounding poor single mothers' union formation and dissolution, with special attention to how these choices met their perceived psychological, emotional, and material needs as they moved through adolescence into emerging and young adulthood and parenthood.

METHODS

Sampling

The sample included 32 women who met the following criteria: age 18 or older; White (self-identified); not currently married or steadily cohabiting; had at least one child; had a very low income; and had attained no formal educational credential beyond a high school diploma or GED. Participation was solicited in and around two small cities in South Carolina through two methods. First, fliers describing the study, including all of the sample inclusion criteria listed above, were placed in waiting areas in two county departments of social services and their welfare-to-work programs. All of the women who responded agreed to participate, and all met the sample inclusion criteria. The second method of recruitment was through snowball sampling. At the end of each interview, we asked the respondent to suggest other women who might be interested in participating in the study.

It is likely that most of the women, many of whom had no steady source of income, participated primarily to earn the $25 that was paid for each interview. This motivation was apparent among several women who agreed to participate contingent upon scheduling the interview, hence receiving payment, within a specified short time, often at the end of the month, when cash tended to be scarce. For example, one woman whose "heart is broken" by the degree to which her poverty and lack of transportation deprive her small son of many pleasures of childhood was anxious to have an interview so that she could get enough money to buy him a Halloween costume. Thus, the financial urgency among these women may represent a sample bias. In addition, using snowball sampling resulted in a few small clusters of respondents within the larger sample who were members of a social and/or kin network. While the majority of respondents knew only one other potential participant, this feature of the sample, the common deep financial need, and the geographical focus on two areas within one state limit generalization of findings.

Data Collection

Data were collected by four researchers—the two authors and two social work doctoral students who had significant experience in clinical practice—over the course of a year-and-a-half. Nearly all interviews took place in the participant's home or current residence, such as the home of a relative or friend, at the discretion of the participant. Interviews were audiotaped and transcribed verbatim.

Data consisted of focused life histories gathered through face-to-face interviews using primarily open-ended questions with active use of probes for detail and clarification. The interview guide provided a set of topics that reflected substantive domains comprising detailed historical and current information about subsistence strategies, including sources of income; housing, including residential movement and physical conditions of current housing; family of origin; educational and occupational experiences and aspirations; marriage and/or cohabitation; their own and their children's relationships with their children's fathers; sexual initiation; pregnancy and motherhood; and hopes for the future of their children and themselves.

Consistent with the inherent nature of qualitative methods in examining individual experience, two major changes were made in the structure and content of the interviews over the course of the study. First, the interviewers became more flexible in guiding the order of topics discussed to accommodate the idiographic way each participant structured her personal life narrative. Second, as reported in other similar research, as unanticipated themes such as domestic violence emerged in early interviews, these themes were explored more explicitly in subsequent interviews (Burton et al., 2001; Bell, 2003; Cherlin et al., 2004).

Data Analysis

The interviews were analyzed in two primary ways: first, thematically across all interviews, using a coding scheme developed by the two authors and a doctoral student who had not conducted any of the interviews and, second, from an individual developmental perspective through constructing a chronological time line for each participant. The qualitative software program NVivo was used to assist in thematic analysis. Like similar programs, NVivo is an efficient means not only for coding interview and other data but for comparing themes within and across subgroups in the sample. The analytic themes were based on categories that were predetermined based upon relevant theory and empirical literature and constituted interview topics and also new themes that emerged from the life histories themselves, such as childhood and adult domestic violence.

RESULTS

Characteristics of the Participants

The age of the 32 participants ranged from 18 to 46. The mean age was 30, but the majority of the women were in their twenties. Over half of the women, 56%, had never been married (referred hereafter as NM). All of the NM participants had lived with a man at least once, their histories ranging from a single relationship to serial cohabitation. Several women had lived with the father(s) of one or more of their children, others only with a boyfriend who had not fathered a child with them, while some had experienced both situations of cohabitation. The remaining 44% of the participants had been married (referred hereafter as EM) and were divorced or separated from their husbands; one woman married at age 15 but annulled it when she discovered her "husband" was already married. Similar to the NM women, most participants who had been married reported complex histories of cohabitation outside of marriage. These cohabiting circumstances included living with their husband or another man before marriage and/or living with a new boyfriend after becoming divorced or separated.

Among the NM women, 56% had two children, 28% had one child, and 16% had three or more children. Half of the EM women had two children, 28% had three or more children, and 22% had one child. Of all of the women with more than one child, 78% experienced multi-partner fertility. Seventy-one percent of NM women had children with different biological fathers, and 57% of EM women had children with more than one man, in a few cases none their husband.

Across the entire sample, the average level of formal education attainted was less than twelfth grade. Among women who had been married, 36% had completed high school; 43% had a GED; and 21% dropped out of high school. A similar proportion of NM women, 33%, graduated from high school, but only 22% went on to earn a GED, and, 44% had less than a high school education. Even within the context of overall low educational attainment, the greater proportion of NM women who dropped out of school is consistent with other studies that find that lower levels of education among women who cohabit than those who marry (Lichter & Qian, 2008).

By definition of eligibility for inclusion in the sample, all of the women, irrespective of their level of educational attainment, were poor in terms of income and other financial assets. Most of the respondents were not living in their "own home" because they could not afford either rent or the deposits necessary to rent most trailers or apartments. Only one woman (NM) and mother of five by age 21, owned her own home, with the help of the father of her three youngest children.

Despite being eligible to receive temporary assistance to needy families (TANF), only 18 women received public welfare benefits in some combination of Medicaid for their children, child care ("ABC") vouchers, and/or food stamps, and only a few received cash assistance. Typically, their sources of cash income were so unreliable that few were able to calculate their annual or even monthly income; among those who could provide specific information, the average was about $8,000 per year—less than the federal poverty line in 2004 for a single individual and about half the poverty line for a family of three. Some women reported having no predictable source of income each month. One NM woman who received "AFDC" (like most other participants she was not aware that TANF had replaced AFDC) and food stamps, expressing the participants' typical situation, reflected that, "It's not enough. We struggle real bad." Another woman, separated from her husband and living with a friend, reported:

> My husband goes to court Thursday. He lost his job, and he's losing his house which is our house. And he's probably going to go to jail ... so, I'm not receiving child support and I really don't have anywhere to live ... the waiting list (for public housing) is a year and I've considered emergency housing because of my situation. They put me in a shelter and I would be there if I didn't my friend, staying here.

At the time of the interview, about 30% of the participants were receiving income from some form of employment, and the remaining women were seeking work. All of the participants had a history of sporadic, low-wage employment. While a few had engaged in prostitution or other illicit means of generating income such as selling drugs, typically their jobs included working as waitresses, in convenience stores, in nursing homes, cleaning houses, babysitting, and the unusual occupation of delivering doves for funerals.

Although the vast majority of the study's 32 participants reached young adulthood with similarly troubled histories of childhood and adolescence, there are a few differences between the women who cohabit but never married and those who have been married. While 57% of EM and 53% of NM women were exposed to domestic violence in their families of origin, almost twice as many—24%—of NM were both victim of and witness to violence during childhood. In terms of their later relationships, 79% of EM participants were victims of domestic violence (by husband and boyfriends) in comparison to 59% of NM participants who were victimized by adult partners.

Another difference among the women in the study is that more NM women report having used drugs and/or alcohol during their adolescent years—71% versus 57% of the EM women. Their marital status does not distinguish the consequences of substance abuse, realized and threatened, such as children being taken into substitute care, mainly by their own family or their babies' fathers or parents, or related criminal charges.

There was little distinction among the women in terms of aspects of partner quality: They overwhelmingly had male partners who engaged in multiple and various kinds of troubled behavior. Most of the women's partners, 79% of husbands and 77% of cohabiting partners, had histories of substance abuse, incarceration and other legal problems, drug trafficking, domestic violence, and/or mental illness. As we see below, these problems were closely interconnected and contributed frequently to the dissolution of their marriages or cohabiting relationships.

Forming and Dissolving Unions: Husbands, Children's Fathers, and Other Partners

Whether men and women marry, cohabit, or divorce is, of course, of greatest significance to the larger society when children are part of the union. For both the EM and NM women in this study, the well-being of their children was central to decisions about relationships with their biological father. These decisions, however, were also influenced by other compelling considerations that are best understood contextually in their individual and familial historical and current circumstances. Most of the women entered into relationships with their children's fathers carrying the emotional, psychological, physical, and economic disadvantages following deeply difficult personal and family histories. A strong majority, 86% of EM and 89% of NM women, reached young adulthood after experiencing multiple forms of emotional and physical trauma, years of growing up rife with some combination of domestic violence, emotional abuse, incest, school failure, poverty, unstable family lives, exposure to and personal use of drugs and alcohol, and early sexual activity and pregnancy (see Farber and Miller-Cribbs, in press for detailed descriptions). The particular configuration of factors for each woman was unique, yet there were overwhelming thematic similarities that highlight their deep interconnectedness over time in motivating any particular act of relational and family formation. The following examination of four women's experiences of marriage and cohabitation together illustrate the predominant elements found among the larger sample of disadvantaged single mothers in the study.

Ever-Married Women

Carrie

At the age of 24, Carrie is the mother of three children—ages, 2, 4, and 6. Carrie is employed, but her income of $100 a week from part-time work as a waitress is "not very much … enough to get by" to support herself and two of her children who live with her. Carrie is especially frustrated by her low income because she needs about $3,000 to pay for a divorce that she hopes to finalize before her husband is released from jail. Although Carrie is anxious to divorce the father of her two younger children, she also is ambivalent about being a single mother because, "I know my kids will grow up without a father and I've done exactly what I didn't want to do. And that's the hardest part for me. Because something I swore I'd never do, I did."

Carrie's views about the importance of marriage and marital childbearing are similar to those of all but two of the EM women in the study who at one time held explicitly high hopes for what a good marriage should be like. Frequently expressed as an ideal of a '50-50' partnership, the women expected husbands to share the financial and practical responsibilities of daily life and be mutually respectful of one another's views and desires. These ideals about marriage are also generally consistent with other findings about the increasingly companionate definition of a marriage and expectations for flexible gender roles among low-income women (Edin and Reed, 2005). Consistent with some other findings about the relative social conservatism of Southern women, Carrie and most of the other married women here also believe that, if possible, children should be born to and live with their married parents. What, then, led Carrie to decisions that appear to conflict so with her stated values about marriage and parenthood?

Though Carrie valued marriage as an ideal and the best context for having children, marriage per se was never a goal for her. After helping her mother plan three of her own five weddings (three to the same man), she concluded, "It's not for me." And marriage was never an option when she first became pregnant at age 16 by Bill, a boy she thought was "the most perfect, sweetest little thing in the world." When she met Bill, she was already living on her own, no longer in her mother's home.

Like Carrie, 57% of the EM participants in the study experienced some form of domestic violence in their families of origin. This included 14% who were childhood victims of physical and/or sexual abuse; 29% who witnessed their mothers being physically abused; and 14% who were both victim and witnesses of physical and/or sexual abuse at home. Carrie was both victim and witness. She ran away from her home frequently after age 12 to escape her step-father's sexual abuse and the severe alcoholism that "drug him down," leaving her mother as sole financial support of the family. Carrie says that "bad things" are all she remembers about her childhood home:

> I remember one night her husband, P., my sister's father, came in and he was drunk and he was ranting and raving as always. And I remember seeing my sister sitting in the corner crying scared and my mother looked over and see how scared she was of her own father.

Although Carrie had met her biological father only once, after neighbors reported suspected abuse by her stepfather, she called her father and went to live with him for a few months. After her mother insisted she return home, Carrie "went into the rebellion thing," was expelled from school, began to spend most of her time with friends, and became sexually active. She returned to a different school, where she was a good student until she met Bill in eleventh grade and become pregnant, something she had always looked forward to to "fill the void" of her loneliness. Carrie immediately dropped out of school and ran away with him. The months of her pregnancy were filled with poor health and emotional crisis. When Carrie finally was admitted to the hospital for severe dehydration, Bill left her there: "He just looked at me and says, 'I'm not ready.' He turned around and walked out of the hospital and I never saw him again." Two years later, Bill joined the military and attempted to gain legal custody of their child. Carrie believed that her young age and poverty put her at risk of losing her son, so her mother and stepfather adopted him but allowed him to continue living with his mother.

Despite Carrie's avowed lack of interest in marrying after witnessing her own mother's difficult marriages, when she met Terry, "It was like nothing else mattered. He was the love of my life." After living together for about one-and-a-half years, Carrie became pregnant. Six months pregnant with her second child, she and Terry got married. She was hopeful for their future together, believing "it was gonna be forever," as marriage should be.

While dating, Carrie knew that Terry was on probation, the result, he told her, of problems with car insurance and a suspended license. Eventually, she discovered that his probation was actually the result of conviction for committing a "lewd lascivious act toward a minor" before they met. However, this discovery came only after a year of marriage during which Carrie's initial expectations for a "forever" life together were shattered. The difference between living together and marriage became apparent to Carrie immediately:

> The first time he ever hit me was the day we got married. He never hit me before we got married. The day we got married, after everyone left and we were getting ready for bed and everything, he just looked at me straight in my eye. He says, "We're married now. You're mine. You'll do whatever I want you to do . . . " He was extremely abusive, alcoholic, drugs, the ranting and raving, the temper.

During their one year of marriage, before Carrie left her husband, she—like 79% of the EM women in this study—experienced chronic and severe domestic violence in at least one adult relationship. For some women here, abuse or its foreshadowing in the form of extreme jealousy began prior to marriage. Most of the women, however, did not face significant physical violence until after they were married, like Tiffany, whose husband developed "this obsession with taking my head and bashing it through the window, mirrors in the bathroom all the time." Other women's husbands made it clear that with marriage came a form of ownership that they were free to express however they chose, including through physical violence and emotional abuse.

As the violence increased, Carrie started working at three jobs to avoid being home, and she made sure that their infant daughter was always at her mother's or a babysitter's home. In order to protect the older child from the violence, Carrie's mother took him to live with her, telling her, "I'm sorry, but you'll understand one day."

A turning point for Carrie came when Terry had a serious car accident with their six-month old daughter, Krystal, in the car. Terry was arrested for DUI and served 2 weeks in jail. Carrie did not attempt to "get him out" and when he returned home, the violence escalated. This upward spiral culminated in the incident that convinced Carrie that, despite being scared to leave Terry, she had to in order to protect her child:

> My daughter was sitting in the living room, and when [Terry] got to the house his buddies were with him.... We were sitting around this huge picnic table playing spades. And all of the sudden, he just picked up the table and throws it on me. Well, I got the table off of me and then we have these barstools that were in between me and him and he went to pick one up. Well, before he did, I picked it up. And I kind of like threw it towards him so I could get by, while he caught it and threw it back at me and hit me with it. Well then, I just grabbed Krystal, I ran out the door, got in the car and left. When I got to the hospital I had three cracked on this side and two broken ribs on this side ... and one of them had bruised my kidney. That was the day I left him. I left everything I had. I just never went back. And he got locked up three weeks later for the violation of probation. It was just the fact that when he threw that barstool I was standing a foot from my daughter. *And it was like it didn't matter to him that she was there, and that was the thing. I was already so upset with what he did in that car with her in there. And I just—my children come before anything else.*

Carrie was pregnant with her third child—their second—when she left her husband, but he has never seen his younger daughter nor does he provide child support for either of their children. In reflecting on the events and choices that brought Carrie to this unplanned state of single motherhood, she understands better her mother's dilemma and remembers when her mother finally left her own abusive husband: "We always knew she wanted to but she would always give in because I guess she didn't want to be alone and that's a problem. I think I'm following in my mother's footsteps."

After what she experienced, Carrie believes she has "grown up" a lot and has a new boyfriend who is kind to her and her children. She would like to get married again to give her children a family but is "real scared" of it. She concludes with the regretful observation that "I just can't eat. I can't do anything. And it's like my nerves are driving me crazy lately. I'm constantly analyzing everything, and it's just things aren't like the way I want them. This isn't what I want."

Darlene

Like Carrie and the other women in the study, Darlene struggles to support herself and her child, 16-month old Tyrell. She is looking for a job but currently relies on public assistance and friends to make ends meet. She has been waiting for over a year to "get a court date" to pursue child support from Jamal, her son's father. Having completed only tenth grade, Darlene's employment options are limited and she must manage her money very carefully: "I'm on a tight budget. You struggle. You have to really learn what priorities are. Food, diapers, wipes, you know, whatever my child needs. That comes first."

Although Darlene loves being a mother and finds parenthood a "good experience," she is "shocked" to find herself being a single mother. This was never her intention, or preference. Darlene's path to single motherhood included marriage but not to the father of her son.

Expressing a common theme among the married participants, Darlene became intimately involved with a man when she was a teenager explicitly because she was "thinking about getting out of my house as fast as I could, any way I could. The first train out, I wanted on it." Most of the other women who suffered domestic abuse as children believe that they developed relationships with their boyfriends as teens, became sexually active, often resulting in teenage pregnancy, in direct response to chaotic and traumatic family situations. Mary expresses this explicit motivation in recounting how she gave up her plan to finish high school and go to college when she married her boyfriend at age 16 as a "ticket out" from her father's extreme violence toward her and her mother and his substance abuse. Echoing Mary's situation, Darlene was both witness to and victim of domestic violence associated with substance abuse in her childhood home:

> I was raised in a very abusive home emotionally, physically. My father just had severe drug and alcohol problems.... He does not work. My mother has always supported him.... I remember him shoving, punching her. He was good at just tearing the house apart. She would beg and cry and plead with him to calm down and to stop. I remember one night, he came home just in this rage and broke everything in the house. The china cabinet, the dishes, the tables, the chairs. And we were in terror. We were in a closet crying and he ended up dragging me and my brother out of the house cussing and screaming at my mother.... And he drove around all night with us in the car in a rage.... I mean that was my dad and I loved him but I didn't want to be with him and I was scared of him.

As Darlene entered adolescence, her father began to "punish" her physically. Although he never made sexual advances to her, she believes that his extreme controlling behavior was a form of sexual jealousy that was checked only by fear that incest "would have been the one thing that might have finally made her [mother] get rid of him." Less fortunate than Darlene, other women suffered ongoing sexual abuse by fathers and other family members. Tracy had sex with the father of her first child at age 14 so that her father wouldn't be the one to "take" her virginity; while Lacey's father, who lived with his parents, "did things to me that he should not have done to me" when she was expected to sleep in the same bed with him.

Between ages 12 and 15, Darlene increasingly became a target of her father's violence, the frequency and severity depending upon his drug use. She began running away regularly and was legally deemed "incorrigible." During these years, Darlene became close to a neighbor, John, 4 years her senior. Darlene sought refuge in their relationship following an explosion of violence perpetrated by her father when she was 15. She "snapped" one night while watching her father talk to her mother about money "like she was a dog":

> I looked at him and told him if he was so Goddamn worried about the bills, why didn't he get off his ass and get a job. And he just kind of immediately jumped up and charged me. Threw me against the wall. Started punching me in the face ... punching me and punching me and punching me.

Darlene defended herself by hitting him with an iron rod, and the melee ended with them both outside, neighbors watching as she screamed for someone to help her and to call the police. No one did, and after Darlene was able to get out of bed the next day, with the help of painkillers, she called John. They immediately went together to a motel, thus beginning 4 years of cohabitation. Unlike the majority of the women's marital and cohabiting partners in this study, John worked steadily, and Darlene had freedom to do what she pleased without worrying about whether "rent was gonna be paid or if my power was gonna be turned off." She was "thrilled" to feel secure with John:

> I was happy and I was safe. I knew he was gonna take care of me. John always took care of me. Because of the way I had grown up in a household where the man didn't take on any responsibility and didn't do the things that he should have done. It was very important to me to have a husband that did that. And John was the complete opposite. He worked all day. Morning to night.

Having dropped out of school and escaped from her nightmarish home situation, Darlene remembers the next several years as a "break" from emotional turmoil, resulting in their decision to marry:

> I think the marriage was a kind of a last-ditch effort to save that relationship because neither one of us wanted to let it go because we had been friends for so long and I was really scared to let him go because ... he was almost like my security blanket because he had taken care of me for so long and I didn't know if I could take care of myself. And I knew with him I never had to worry about bills or anything. I was never gonna have to worry about any of the stuff that I had to worry about growing up.

Marriage satisfied their mutual needs until John became more and more "possessive":

> Initially it was a really, really good relationship I thought. John really—he definitely loved me but he loved me too much. He wanted to be with me 24 hours a day. And of course that was great and wonderful because, you know, I'm a 16-year old girl.... But eventually as I got a little bit older and a little bit more confident, and I wanted to become a little more independent, he was not happy with that. He didn't want me to really have friends after a while ...

As the tension between Darlene's growing need for independence and John's desire to keep the original balance in their relationship grew, they became sexually and emotionally estranged. Finally, during one of their increasingly frequent arguments, John tried to take Darlene's car keys and credit cards and slapped her in the face, evidence to her that he had "turned into" her controlling and abusive father. She immediately filed a police report and left her husband, keeping her promise that, "I was never gonna be hit by a man. Never."

Contributing to John's anger was suspicion that Darlene was having an affair. Indeed, toward the end of their marriage, Darlene met and began a casual relationship with Jamal, who was a correctional officer at a prison. She was immediately attracted to him and especially taken with the fact that he was a devoted father to his baby, with whose mother he had no ongoing relationship. After Darlene left John, she and Jamal began living together and began trying to have a baby. After Darlene became pregnant, however, the qualities that had drawn her to Jamal—his "sweetness" with his baby and employment stability—evaporated. Darlene discovered that, in fact, he was a "spoiled, self-centered man.... It's just in his instinct for him to think of himself first. Not his children, not his mother, not anyone else." Even though her pregnancy was planned, Jamal became less and less involved over the months. When he quit his job, during the seventh month of her pregnancy, Darlene left Jamal:

> I was tired of just Jamal being feeling like he was number one. He was just inconsiderate. Like he wouldn't clean or he wouldn't cook or he wouldn't go to the doctor's appointments with me. He made me feel like he didn't care anymore ... and then when he quit his job and that said to me he didn't care about our child that was the last straw for me.

Jamal worked again for a while before their son was born, and Darlene moved back in with him. Soon after their second try at cohabitation, Jamal became a "dominant man," insisting that Darlene cook and clean to his satisfaction; and he was not responsible about paying their bills. She observes that he never hit her, but the constant conflict became intolerable. Unwilling to submit to feeling controlled and remain with a man who, like her father, was not financially stable, Darlene left Jamal.

> I think he thought that when I got this apartment I was gonna be, like "Come on down and move in." And when he saw that that wasn't gonna happen he's just got really antagonistic. I don't want to be

with him. I just—I can't see that working out. I want him to be involved in his son's life. But as far as my life, no. I have no desire to be with him.

As Darlene reflects on her current circumstances, she observes that although she had "made bad decisions ... getting involved with the men I did and just kind of stuck," she likely would have made the same decisions again because of her desperation to leave her parents' house. Darlene hopes to attain her GED and then to leave South Carolina because of the risks of raising her son who, like several of the other participants' children, is biracial, in such an unpromising environment:

> I look at all these men here not working and especially in this neighborhood. Not working and drinking and drugging and I don't feel like this is a good environment. And a lot of racism and he's a bi-racial child.... And so you know this (TANF) class is full of single mothers and we're all dealing with it. You know we're not getting child support. The fathers aren't there. They're in jail or they're wherever and [we're] just kind of left to fend for ourselves and our children.

Never-Married Women

Although there are some differences among the EM and NM women, as described above, the themes that suffuse the years of their childhood and young adulthood and subsequent choices of partners are more alike than dissimilar. This is evident in the experiences of never-married women, Kayla and Cheryl, described below.

Kayla

Kayla, age 27, does not like to depend on public assistance or her family to help support her 8- and 2-year old daughters, which still leaves her with "nothing hardly" to provide for their needs. However, with only a ninth-grade education and no financial support from the girls' father, Steve, she does not have many good alternative sources of income. Despite the hardships of unmarried motherhood, Kayla feels sure that that she and her children are better than if she had married their father, that marrying Steve "would have been a bigger mistake than leaving school."

Kayla, like about a third of the NM women here and consistent with other findings about poor women's attitudes, does not believe that there is a necessary connection between being married and having children. Joanne expresses Kayla's and others' view that marriage to a child's father represents a distinct form of commitment from that of motherhood because, "if I was married to him, that would be two things.... If we were married, that's a big thing. You also kind of think to get a marriage undone is really complicated compared to just walking away."

Early in their relationship, Kayla decided she would never marry Steve because he cheated on her. However, she continued to live with him because she told herself, "He won't do it no more." The birth of their first child during that first year of living together increased Kayla's commitment to their relationship:

> I had a kid, and it wasn't because of her, I mean not all of it. Yeah, some of it is because we had a kid together, and you know, I figured, let's try to make it work. I tried my best to make it work, and swallowed my pride....

When Kayla met Steve, she had already dropped out of school, something she now regards as the biggest mistake she has made. She had always been a poor student, and one day tenth grade, decided not to go back because she "hated" it and was "wasting" her time when she could be "out partying or riding, cruising, whatever, like normal kids." When Kayla was 14, her parents' divorce had a "bad impact" on her. In the wake of the family's disruption, she became depressed and "got in trouble a lot":

> It was a very, very, very rough divorce. Well, you grow up your whole live in the church and not believing in divorce and then all of a sudden, whammy, it hits you. If both of your parents separate, you have to choose, and both them started smoking, both of them started drinking, they quit going to church, so therefore I started learning the different life, and I sort of took that road then.

After leaving school, Kayla worked at a fast-food restaurant and felt she was "doing good" in having her own trailer and car. When she and Steve met, he immediately moved in with her. Kayla soon broke up with Steve and had a brief relationship with his cousin who severely physically abused her. She returned to Steve, continuing what became a 10-year relationship with the father of her two children. She believed that, at the age of 19, she had found the "man of my dreams . . . We're going to have a child, we're going to have a car . . . and we're going to have a house and a swing set and a front porch." As an expression of faith that she would achieve that "dream," Kayla planned her first pregnancy. However, little about Kayla's life with Steve matched the "picture" in her mind. Instead, ". . . everything just started going downhill, and it never changed after that. Pretty much stayed downhill. It was that longest downhill I ever went down." That "downhill" included years of economic and emotional instability in their growing family:

> He moved in with me, and then I got pregnant with M. I had to quit my job. He said he was going to pay the bills, he didn't, we lost our first trailer, and I lost my car. I lost everything financially because of him—my credit's ruined. . . . We moved in with his mom over in X Trailer Park—terrible place to live—with all of his family and all of his family's friends and their girlfriends and their girlfriends' friends. Well, I hated it. It wasn't a very good lifestyle to live, but he was used to it because that's how he was raised.

Over the ensuing years, the turmoil in their lives increased. By the time Kayla was pregnant a third time—her second unplanned conception, the previous one ending in a stillbirth—they had had two trailers repossessed and had no car. Steve, who continued to work only sporadically, "got real bad on drugs and spent all his money up and didn't never pay the bills."

As Steve's drug use escalated, including crack, he began to be physically violent toward Kayla. She left him more than once but always returned when he promised to treat her better. The last time they reconciled, Steve worked for a while, and Kayla was optimistic, but the changes were short-lived. It was Steve's lack of financial responsibility that finally convinced Kayla that their relationship was not worth the many costs of staying with him:

> Then all of the sudden everything comes crashing back down again and we was . . . nine months behind on our trailer payment . . . I ended up being the only one working, bartending. He wouldn't work. I didn't really get paid a whole lot of money, not enough to pay a trailer payment and land payment, so I left, and now it's better being without him. I'm not living with my parents. I have my license. I'm fixing to get me a car. He doesn't have any of that. He's not even trying to better hisself. I couldn't take it anymore. He was driving me crazy . . .

Kayla regrets that her children do not have a real "daddy," somebody who is really "there" for them, as she remembers her own father in earlier times. However, she does not think that she will get married unless she finds someone who is different from all of the men she has been involved with because, "Every man I've ever dated . . . has cheated on me, and they've all treated me like crap. I mean—I let them." Her current boyfriend seems to be caring toward her and her children, and, "He hasn't cheated on me yet."

Cheryl

The father of Cheryl's younger child, age 2, did not acknowledge paternity until their daughter was a year old. Similar to the many low-income unmarried fathers who experience serial and multi-partner fertility, Rick has children with another woman with whom he lives (Manlove, Logan, Ikramullah, & Holbombe, 2008). Despite Rick's current girlfriend's efforts to limit his sharing financial and emotional resources with Cheryl and the child he shares with her, Cheryl is one of only a few women in the study to receive any child support. Not having to "depend on a man" is an important value for Cheryl. However, it is very difficult to find employment, with only a GED, that is "gonna be able to work with your schedule and what happens if a child gets sick ... and you don't have somebody that could stay home with the kids."

Independence has been a constant theme throughout Cheryl's chaotic life. Echoing many of the women in the study, Cheryl's main aspiration throughout her childhood was "just to get away" from her parents. Cheryl's parents divorced when she was 10, ending a family life characterized by poverty, and domestic violence that occurred "just when they were drinking":

> Well, they drank every night.... I sat in my bedroom many, many nights and cried myself to sleep. I watched my dad stomp on my mom one night when he came in drunk and broke her collar bone. And he wouldn't let us leave the house and she had to crawl into the car and drive herself to the hospital.... And that was one night that I remember just starting to hate my dad.... I remember growing up in dumpy trailers and not being able to walk around in them because there are so much clothes and just filth everywhere.

After the divorce, Cheryl "floated back and forth between mom and dad." This "floating" led Cheryl to run away frequently to avoid her father's physical violence toward her and her mother's alcoholic deterioration:

> Mom stayed in the bars. I took care of her. Watched her. We did whatever we wanted to. Well, my dad's never really been there for me and my mom, she's always kind of drifting away.... So basically I had to do everything on my own.

Cheryl began drinking heavily at 14. Concerned about the "partying" that Cheryl and her siblings engaged in, their aunt finally intervened by calling the police, and "that's how we got into foster care and they charged my mom with neglect and she just, she ran."

Cheryl was placed first with foster parents and then, at age 16, into an independent living program. By the time she was 17 and emancipated from foster care, she had "started to straighten up from the stuff that I was doing, like running the roads, running away from shelters and kind of rebelling against my foster parents, smoking pot, drinking, whatever."

Cheryl met Charles, the father of her first child, just a couple of weeks after she left the independent living program, at the restaurant where she worked: "I had all these facial piercings and he comes to the cash register and he looked at me and he said, 'You're shiny.' He got my phone number and then he like moved in. He never left."

Cheryl became pregnant quickly, but miscarried. She thought their relationship was "wonderful" until discovering that Charles had been having sexual relations with several of her friends since the miscarriage. He broke up with her, he explained, because she had gained weight during her pregnancy. After reconciling, Cheryl and Charles purchased a trailer, had a child, and continued to cohabitate off and on. Their relationship was punctuated regularly by mutual accusations of infidelity, which were not unfounded.

Another constant in their relationship was tension over Charles forbidding Cheryl from working except for helping her father, with whom she had reestablished a connection. Cheryl interprets Charles' desire to control her employment as a way to keep her from having enough money of her own to be independent of him. This effort to control her began to be expressed through physical violence. In one particularly dangerous attack, Charles "picked me up and swung me up against the wall with [the baby] in my arms."

During a period in which Cheryl and Charles were "separated but still living together," she had a sexual relationship with an old friend, Rick, and "ended up pregnant" with his child. Her relationship with Charles ended, and he is not in contact with their son. Charles is expecting a child with his current girlfriend. Cheryl has a new relationship with Jack, who has "never really held a steady job or had a driver's license," but was always "supportive" during the time before Rick became involved in their child's life. She trusts and feels safe with Jack, but because he is "locked up—burglary charge," she does not know what their future holds.

Cheryl was diagnosed with bipolar disorder as a teenager but believes that the doctors "really messed up" that assessment, that what she suffers from is "nerves" from the lifelong stress she has faced. Amid the complicated relationships and economic hardships Cheryl continues to experience, she loves being a mother and is happy to be free from Charles:

> I don't feel like I have to depend on a man and that's always been a big issue for me. I wanted to work but it was always something that came along so I felt like I had to depend on Charles and he kept throwing it up in my face—it's his money, it's his house, because he pays for it. I don't like that. I don't want to depend on anybody. I enjoy living me and my kids. That's all that matters to me. And it's hard and it has trying times, but it's, you know, it's worth it.

DISCUSSION

The life history data from our study of 32 poor White single mothers in the non-metro South reveal complex patterns of instability in formation and dissolution of marital and cohabiting unions. The women's narratives about their relationships with men explicitly include reference to factors identified in other research about barriers to marriage among poor women such as male unemployment, multi-partnered fertility, expectation of companionate marriage, and intolerance of maltreatment. However, this study also suggests an important caveat to the prevailing categorical distinctions between poor women who marry and those who cohabit that supports the analytic framework of Cherlin et al. (2004) focusing on whether unions are stable or transitory among women who have experienced domestic violence. Both the EM and NM women experienced high levels of childhood trauma and poverty in their families of origin; and this trauma was associated with psychological, emotional, social, educational, economic, and other disadvantages that influenced their choices, at young ages, of troubled partners in both marital and cohabitating unions. The vulnerabilities originating in childhood built, one upon the other, leaving the women at heightened risk of relationship difficulties, physical, and mental health problems, compromised parenting and other sources of stress faced by many poor women. Both the vulnerabilities associated with childhood domestic violence, sexual abuse, and other forms of family chaos and their impact in terms of restricted life options and partner choice that dominate the narratives of both NM and EV married women suggest no simple calculation accounted for their decisions about romantic partnerships. Rather, most often ostensibly, they were seeking emotional and economic shelter in relationships with men.

Consistent with the conclusion of Lichter et al. (2003) that marriage is not, in crucial ways, a "panacea" for poor unwed mothers, there is no evidence in these women's life histories that marriage served to mediate their vulnerability in the present or the future. In fact, for some women, marriage was a legally sanctioned trap that exposed both their children and themselves to physical and psychological danger. Building on the findings of Arata & Lindman (2002), many of the women in this study left home early to escape domestic abuse, often sexual in nature, and married or began cohabiting at a young age, only to find themselves re-victimized by their adult partners.

The early experiences with domestic violence and substance abuse in their families of origin were, by the women's own accounts, often connected to their own adolescent patterns of using drugs and alcohol and abridged educational attainment. Subsequent involvement with abusive and substance-abusing men further diminished their educational and vocational attainment and thus their capacity for financial independence. The women's choices grew ever more limited over time as they struggled to protect and support their children.

Certain characteristics of rural life may exacerbate the consequences we find here that are associated with domestic violence among both the married and cohabiting women. Lack of transportation, child care and shelters, geographic and social isolation, higher incidence of weapons in the household, limited access to health care services, limited social services, job opportunities, and training all contribute to the difficulties these and many other rural women face in their attempts to leave violent and abusive relationships (Johnson & O'Brien-Strain, 2000).

Our study suggests that disadvantaged young women whose early lives have left them vulnerable to engaging in romantic relationships with men who are poor prospects as adult partners and fathers might have benefited from early intervention focused on reducing their high-risk behavior and disengagement from school that contributed to such limited alternatives in the context of abusive partnerships. At the same time, if we are concerned about the decline in stable, long-term unions among the poor, we may need to consider measures that would directly reduce the high levels of physical and sexual abuse that women must bear.

RECOMMENDATIONS

Several policy and programmatic implications as well as directions for future research follow from the findings reported here. Overall, policies should be more responsive to the particular circumstances of poor women who experience abuse. For example, given the greater vulnerability of poor women to domestic abuse, it is important to heighten awareness of how the "Family Violence Options" that are a part of TANF may affect these women and their children who are at risk. Many states currently have or are considering policies that automatically link child abuse with domestic violence. However, given what we know about the dynamics of domestic violence in the lives of poor women, policies should encourage greater caution in using child protective service interventions automatically in situations of domestic violence. Instead services should be geared to help women safely remove themselves and their children from violence.

Given the growing body of evidence that demonstrates an association between adverse childhood experiences and later health behaviors and health/mental health outcomes, practitioners working with vulnerable women should assess these adverse experiences and their relationship to current experiences of violence and trauma as they deploy intervention strategies at the micro-level, particularly those aimed at marriage promotion. On a larger scale, policies that account for variability in experiences within marriage as opposed to a blanket approach to marriage promotion are warranted. As this paper and other research suggests, marriage is not a panacea for women and indeed may be a source of risk for some subsets of women in perpetuating circumstances that create vulnerability to interpersonal violence. When women experience interpersonal violence, it is often difficult for them to reach economic self-sufficiency due to job interruption and disruption and, when these women have children, they may risk exposing their children to abuse.

Future research that examines the developmental impacts of traumatic events across the lifespan will continue to inform intervention strategies at both the micro- and macro-levels and for women, men, and their children. Further, research that evaluates the efficacy of marriage promotion programs that account for the impacts of marriage in the context of varying demographic factors and the experience of adverse childhood experiences are also needed.

REFERENCES

Arata, C. M. (2000). From child victim to adult victim: A model for predicting sexual revictimization. *Child Maltreatment*, *5*(1), 28–38.

Arata, C. M., & Lindman, L. (2002). Marriage, child abuse, and sexual revictimization. *Journal of Interpersonal Violence*, *17*(9), 953–968.

Becker, G. S. (1981). *A treatise on the family*. Cambridge, MA: Harvard University Press.

Bell, H. (2003). Cycles within cycles. *Violence Against Women*, *9*(10), 1245–1262.

Blackwell, D., & Lichter, D. (2000). Mate selection among married and cohabiting couples. *Journal of Family Issues*, *21*, 275–302.

Boney-McCoy, S., & Finkelhor, D. (1996). Is youth victimization related to trauma symptoms and depression after controlling for prior symptoms and family relationships? A longitudinal, prospective study. *Journal of Consulting and Clinical Psychology*, *64*(6), 1406–1416.

Briere, J. (1992). *Child abuse trauma: Theory and treatment of lasting effects*. Newbury Park, CA: Sage.

Brown, S., Sanchez, L., Nock, S., & Wright, J. (2006). Links between premarital cohabitation and subsequent marital quality, stability, and divorce: A comparison of covenant versus standard marriages. *Social Science Research*, *35*, 454–470.

Bumpass, L., & Lu, H. (2000). Trends in cohabitation and implications for children's family contexts in the United States. *Population Studies*, *54*, 29–41.

Burton, L. M., Jarrett, R., Lein, L., Mathews, S., Quane, J., & Skinner, D. (2001, April). Structured discovery: Ethnography, welfare reform, and the assessment of neighborhoods, families, and children. Paper presented at the Biennial Meeting of the Society for Research in Child Development, Minneapolis, MN.

Cherlin, A. J., Burton, L. M., Hurt, T. R., & Purvin, D. M. (2004, Dec). The influence of physical and sexual abuse on marriage and cohabitation. *American Sociological Review*, *69*, 768–789.

Cicchetti, D., & Blender, J. (2004, Dec 14). A multiple level analysis approach to the study of developmental processes in maltreated children. *Proceedings of the National Academy of Science*, *101*(50), 17325–17326.

Cloitre, M., Tardiff, K., Marzuk, P. M., Leon, A. C., & Portera, L. (1996). Childhood abuse and subsequent sexual assault among female inpatients. *Journal of Traumatic Stress*, *9*(3), 473–482.

Cohan, C. L., & Bradbury, T. N. (1997). Negative life events, marital interactions, and the longitudinal course of newlywed marriage. *Journal of Personality and Social Psychology*, *73*, 114–128.

Crnic, K. A., & Acevedo, M. (1995). Everyday stress in parenting. In M. H. Bornstein (Ed.), *Handbook of parenting* (1st ed., pp. 277–297). Mahwah, NJ: Lawrence Erlbaum Associates.

Currie, J., & Stabile, M. (2006). Child mental health and human capital accumulation: The case of ADHD. *Journal of Health Economics*, *25*(6), 1094–1118.

Davis, J. L., & Petretic-Jackson, P. A. (2000). The impact of child sexual abuse on adult interpersonal functioning: A review and synthesis of the empirical literature. *Aggression and Violent Behavior*, *5*(3), 291–328.

DeKlyen, M., Brooks-Gunn, J., McLanahan, S., & Knab, J. (2006). The mental health of married, co-habitating, and non-coresident parents with infants. *American Journal of Public Health*, *96*(10), 1836–1841.

DiLillo, D. (2001). Interpersonal functioning among women reporting a history of childhood sexual abuse: Empirical findings and methodological issues. *Clinical Psychology Review*, *21*, 553–576.

Edin, K. (2000). What do low-income single mothers say about marriage? *Social Problems*, *47*(1), 112–133.

Edin, K., & Kefalas, M. (2005). *Promises I can keep*. Berkeley, CA: University of California Press.

Edin, K., & Reed, J. (2005). Why don't they just get married? Barriers to marriage among the disadvantaged. *Marriage and Child Wellbeing*, *15*(2), 117–137.

Edward, W. A., Gelfand, A., Katon, W. J., Koss, M. P., Korff, M. V., Bernstein, D., ... Russo, J. (1999). Adult health status of women with histories of childhood abuse and neglect. *The American Journal of Medicine*, *107*(4), 332–338.

Ellwood, D. T., & Jencks, C. (2006). The spread of single-parent families in the United States since 1960. In D. P. Moynihan, T. M. Smeeding, & L. Rainwater (Eds.), *The future of the family*. New York, NY: Russell Sage Foundation.

Farber, N., & Miller-Cribbs, J. (in press). Violence in the lives of rural, southern and poor white women. *Violence Against Women*.

Fergusson, D. M., Horwood, J. L., & Lynskey, M. T. (1997). Childhood sexual abuse, adolescent sexual behaviors, and sexual revictimization. *Child Abuse & Neglect*, *21*(8), 789–803.

Finkelhor, D., Hotaling, G., Lewis, I. A., & Smith, C. (1989). Sexual abuse and its relationship to later sexual satisfaction, marital status, religion, and attitudes. *Journal of Interpersonal Violence, 4*(4), 379–399.

Gibson-Davis, C. M., Edin, K., & McLanahan, S. (2005, December). High hopes but even higher expectations: The retreat from marriage among low-income couples. *Journal of Marriage and Family, 67*, 1301–1312.

Gidycz, C. A., Hanson, K., & Layman, M. J. (1995). A prospective analysis of the relationships among sexual assault experiences. *Psychology of Women Quarterly, 19*(1), 5–29.

Goldstein, J. R., & Kenney, C. T. (2001, August). Marriage delayed or marriage forgone? New cohort forecasts of first marriage for U.S. women. *American Sociological Review, 66*, 506–519.

Harknett, K., & McLanahan, S. S. (2004). Racial and ethnic differences in marriage after the birth of a child. *American Sociological Review, 69*, 790–811.

Himelein, M. J. (1995). Risk factors for sexual victimization in dating. *Psychology of Women Quarterly, 19*(1), 31–48.

Jasinski, J. (2004). Pregnancy and domestic violence: A review of the literature. *Trauma Violence Abuse, 4*(47), 47–54. Retrieved from http://www.hawaii.edu/hivandaids/Pregnancy_and_Domestic_Violence_A_Review_of_the_Literature.pdf

Johnson, H. P., & O'Brien-Strain, M. (2000). Getting to know the future customers of the Office of Child Support Projections Report for 2004 and 2009. Retrieved from http://www.acf.hhs.gov/programs/cse/pubs/reports/projections/index.html

Kia-Keating, M., Sorsoli, L., & Grossman, F. K. (2009). Relational challenges and recovery processes in male survivors of childhood sexual abuse. *Journal of Interpersonal Violence, 25*(4), 666–681.

Liang, B., Williams, L. M., & Siegel, J. A. (2006). Relational outcomes of childhood sexual trauma in female survivors: A longitudinal study. *Journal of Interpersonal Violence, 21*(1), 42–57.

Lichter, D. T., & Graefe, D. R. (2007). Men and marriage promotion: Who marries unmarried mothers? *Social Service Review, 81*(3), 397–421.

Lichter, D. T., Graefe, D. R., & Brown, J. B. (2003). Is marriage a panacea? Union formation among economically disadvantaged unwed mothers. *Social Problems, 50*(1), 60–86.

Lichter, D. T., & Qian, Z. (2008, Nov). Serial cohabitation and the marital life course. *Journal of Marriage and Family, 70*, 861–878.

Lichter, D. T., Qian, Z., & Mellott, L. M. (2006, May). Marriage or dissolution? Union transitions among poor cohabiting women. *Demography, 43*(2), 223–240.

Manlove, J., Logan, C., Ikramullah, E., & Holcombe, E. (2008, May). Factors associated with multiple-partner fertility among fathers. *Journal of Marriage and Family, 70*(2), 536–548.

Manning, W. D., & Smock, P. J. (2005). Measuring and modeling cohabitation: New perspectives form qualitative data. *Journal of Marriage and Family, 67*, 989–1002.

Moore, K., Redd, Z., Burkhauser, M., Mbwana, K., & Collins, A. (2009). *Children in poverty: Trends, consequences, and policy options* (Research Brief No. 2009-11). Washington, DC: Child Trends. Retrieved from http://www.childtrends.org/files/child_trends-2009_04_07_rb_childreninpoverty.pdf

Nelson, B. S., & Wampler, K. S. (2000). Systematic effects of trauma in clinic couples: An exploratory study of secondary trauma resulting from childhood abuse. *Journal of Marital and Family Therapy, 26*(2), 171–184.

Raley, R. K., & Bumpass, L. (2003). The topography of the divorce plateau: Levels and trends in union stability in the United States after 1980. *Demographic Research, 8*, 245–260. doi: 10.4054/DemRes.2003.8.8

Randall, A. & Bodenmann, G. (2009). The role of stress on close relationships and marital satisfaction. *Clinical Psychology Review, 29*(2), 105–115.

Reed, J. (2007). Anatomy of the breakup. In P. England & K. Edin (Eds.), *Unmarried couples with children* (pp. 133–156). New York, NY: Russell Sage Foundation.

Rumstein-McKean, O., & Hunsley, J. (2001). Interpersonal and family functioning of female survivors of childhood sexual abuse. *Clinical Psychology Review, 21*(3), 471–490.

Seltzer, J. A. (2000, November). Families formed outside of marriage. *Journal of Marriage and Family, 62*(4), 1247–1268.

Smock, P. J. (2000). Cohabitation in the United States: An appraisal of research themes, findings, and implications. *Annual Review of Sociology, 26*, 1–20.

Smock, P. J., Manning, W. D., & Porter, M. (2005). Everything's there except money: How money shapes decisions to marry among cohabitors. *Journal of Marriage and the Family, 5I3*(3), 680–696.

Solomon-Fears, C. (2008). Nonmarital childbearing: Trends, reasons, and public policy interventions. Congressional Research Service (U.S.), November 20, 2008. Report No. RL34756. Retrieved from http://www.fas.org/sgp/crs/misc/RL34756.pdf

Teitler, J. O., & Reichman, N. E. (2001, March). Cohabitation: An elusive concept. Paper presented at the Annual Meeting of the Population Association of America, Washington, DC.

Teitler, J. O., & Reichman, N. E. (2008). Mental illness as a barrier to marriage among unmarried mothers. *Journal of Marriage and Family, 70*(3), 772–782.

Waldfogel, J., Craigie, T., & Brooks-Gunn, J. (2010). Fragile families and child well-being. *Fragile Families*, *20*(2), 87–112. Retrieved from http://futureofchildren.org/publications/journals/article/index.xml?journalid=73&articleid=532&sectionid=3659

Webster-Stratton, C. (1990). Stress: A potential disruptor of parent perceptions and family interactions. *Journal of Clinical Child Psychology*, *19*(4), 302–312.

Whelan, R. (1994). *Broken homes and battered children*. Marsh Barton, Exeter, UK: Family Education Trust.

Whisman, M. A. (2006). Childhood trauma and marital outcomes in adulthood. *Personal Relationships*, *13*(4), 375–386.

Wilson, W. J. (1987). *The truly disadvantaged: The inner city, the underclass, and public policy*. Chicago, IL: The University of Chicago Press.

Wind, T. W., & Silvern, L. (1992). Type and extent of child abuse as predictors of adult functioning. *Journal of Family Violence*, *7*, 216–281.

Wu, L. (2008, Feb). Cohort estimates of nonmarital fertility for U.S. women. *Demography*, *45*(1), 193–207.

Wu, L., Bumpass, L., & Musick, K. (2001). Stability of marital and cohabitating unions following a first birth. In L. L. Wu & B. Wolfe (Eds.), *Out of wedlock: Causes and consequences of nonmarital fertility* (pp. 3–48). New York, NY: Russell Sage Foundation.

African American Marital Satisfaction as a Function of Work-Family Balance and Work-Family Conflict and Implications for Social Workers

Noelle M. St. Vil

Department of Community and Public Health, Johns Hopkins School of Nursing, Baltimore, Maryland, USA

African Americans are more likely than any other race/ethnic group to report lower levels of marital satisfaction. Due to numerous benefits of marriage such as better physical and mental health, it is important to identify factors that impact African American marital satisfaction. This study examines the impact of work-family conflict and work-family balance on African American marital satisfaction. The results reveal a negative relationship between work-family conflict and marital satisfaction as well as differences in work-family factors that predict husbands' verses wives' marital satisfaction. The article offers implications for social work.

Benefits to marriage include better economic, physical, and mental health, as well as a better overall quality of life compared to those who are not married. Despite benefits to marriage, marriage rates have been on the decline since the 1970s (Teachman, Tedrow, & Crowder, 2000). While 85% of the U.S. population will marry at least once (U.S. Bureau of the Census, 2006), the average couple who marries has a 40% to 50% chance of experiencing divorce or separation (Wilcox, Marquardt, Popnoe, & Whitehead, 2009). Proponents of the marital decline perspective, those who believe that personal happiness has become more important than marriage obligations (Loveless & Holman, 2007), attribute high divorce rates to the belief that it has become difficult to maintain satisfied marriages (Amato, Booth, & Johnson, 2003). Marital satisfaction refers to a global assessment of the quality of an individual's marriage according to one's internal chosen criteria. An individual weighs perceived costs and benefits of his or her marriage. If perceived benefits outweigh perceived costs, then an individual will report having a satisfied marriage; however, if perceived costs outweigh perceived benefits, an individual will report being in a dissatisfied marriage (Stone & Shackelford, 2007).

Studies reveal that overall, African Americans report experiencing lower levels of marital satisfaction than other races (Broman, 1993, 2002, 2005; Bulanda & Brown, 2008; Trent & South, 2003). African American women experience lower marital satisfaction compared to African American males (Bulanda & Brown, 2008; Lincoln & Chae, 2010) and their White (Broman, 1993; Trent & South, 2003), Hispanic (Bulanda & Brown, 2008), and Afro Caribbean (Bryant, Taylor,

Lincoln, Chatters, & Jackson, 2008) male and female counterparts. In addition, African Americans have lower rates of marriage and marital stability than all other ethnic groups (Administration of Child and Families, 2006) and African Americans are more likely to think about getting a divorce (Broman, 2002). Racial differences in levels of marital satisfaction are unexplained (Trent & South, 2003). In order to promote lasting and healthy marriages, it is important to identify factors that impact African American martial satisfaction. In a society where dual earner families are increasing and more spouses are confronted with the task of juggling both work and family, two factors that warrant further study is work-family balance and work-family conflict and its impact on marital satisfaction.

WORK-FAMILY BALANCE AND WORK-FAMILY CONFLICT

Work-family balance perceives work-family relationships as compatible. The expectations of work combined with the expectations of family create an enriching experience that is characterized by accomplishments in balancing roles and responsibilities of the work realm with the family realm (Grzwacz & Carlson, 2007). The experiences in one role, work or family, enhances the experiences in the other role (Gareis, Barnett, Ertel, & Berkman, 2009). The two roles are complementary.

Work-family conflict perceives work-family relationships as the incongruence of an individual's work demands and an individual's family demands. When demands from work and family are mutually incompatible, inter-role conflict is created (Greenhaus & Beutell, 1985). The belief is that the work and family realm cannot coexist but rather must be balanced with one domain receiving higher priority than the other (Byron, 2005). The literature identifies work-family conflict as being bidirectional (Bianchi & Milkie, 2010; Hughes & Parks, 2007; Voyandoff, 2005), meaning it includes work-to-family conflict and family-to-work conflict (Gareis et al., 2009). Work-to-family conflict results in work expectations interfering or conflicting with family domain while family-to-work results in family expectations interfering with the work domain (Tatman, Hovestadt, Yelsma, Fenell, & Canfield, 2006). Work-to family conflict is viewed as arising from job conditions, and family-to-work conflict arises from conditions in the home (Bianchi & Milkie, 2010).

How individuals manage and perceive work and family roles may have major implications for marital satisfaction. For example, a wife and mother who works full-time may receive a call from her child's school during work hours stating that her child is not feeling well. She calls her husband to see whether he is able to tend to their child. However, he is in a meeting, so she must once again sacrifice her time at work in order to address family needs. This could lead to resentment toward her husband if she feels she is the only one in the marriage making an effort to balance both family and life roles. In addition, a father, husband, and employee may try to excel in both his work and family roles but feels his primary role is to monetarily support the family, so he spends most of his time at work and less time with the family. This could lead to friction between the husband and wife.

WORK-FAMILY BALANCE, WORK-FAMILY CONFLICT, AND MARITAL SATISFACTION

Literature has shown that perceptions of work-family conflict lead to lower martial satisfaction (Mitchelson, 2009) and increases in divorce (Hammer & Thompson, 2003). For example, Kossek and Ozeki (1998) found that regardless of direction, work-to-family or family-to-work, a consistent negative relationship existed between work-family conflict and job-life satisfaction. Similarly, Barnett, Campo, Campo, and Steiner (2003) in their study of work-family balance among Mexican

Americans found that individuals who perceived higher levels of work-family balance reported higher levels of marital quality and vice versa. In addition, a qualitative study conducted by Wong and Goodwin (2009) across three cultures (London, Hong Kong, and Beijing) found that one-third of individuals reported a negative interference of work on their marriage. The three cultures examined were all modernized societies where both individuality and intimate relationships are emphasized. This is similar to African Americans living in American culture who are influenced by a culture that promotes individuality but yet has its roots in a culture that promotes kinship and community. The conflicting messages from multiple cultural values make it difficult to prioritize and balance work and family realms.

The majority of research conducted in the area of work-family balance has consisted of Anglo-American samples (Barnett et al., 2003). The same holds true for research conducted on marital satisfaction (Bryant et al., 2008). Overall, research pertaining to African Americans, marital satisfaction and work-family balance is scarce. Since African Americans report the lowest levels of marital satisfaction compared to other racial and ethnic groups, it is important to identify factors that contribute to marital satisfaction. The identification of factors such as work-family balance is crucial in meeting the marriage and family needs of African Americans.

Due to the benefits of marriage and the established relationship of the effects of work-family balance and work-family conflict on marital satisfaction, social workers are likely to be confronted with couples experiencing these issues. The results of this study will yield social work implications that may adequately prepare social workers to provide effective services when working with African American couples and work and family issues. For example, in order to effectively assist African Americans in balancing work and family, studies must be conducted in which the outcomes are compared with the findings of the mainstream; if outcomes are similar, then existing methods of assisting couples in balancing work and family may be relevant. However, if outcomes differ, culturally competent and gender-specific practices will need to be adopted in assisting African Americans with work-family balance.

This study seeks to examine the relationship between work-family balance, work-family conflict, and marital satisfaction of African Americans. The results of the study will yield social work implications so that social workers can better assist African Americans in managing work and family, which can increase marital satisfaction. In order to expand the expertise of the social worker to the marriage realm, I will begin by proposing ways that social workers can effectively work with African American couples to balance their work and family life so that the benefits of marital satisfaction are received by all the individuals in the family.

This study seeks to answer two research questions:

(1) What is the impact of work-family balance and work-family conflict on African American marital satisfaction?
(2) Do the work-family balance and work-family conflict variables that best predict African American marital satisfaction differ by gender?

DATA AND METHODS

Sample

This secondary analysis utilizes data from the Married and Cohabitating 2010 [United States] data set, which is a study that was conducted by the National Center for Marriage & Family Research at Bowling Green State University. Data consisted of a nationally representative sample of U.S. married and cohabitating adults between the ages of 18 and 64. In order to answer the research questions in this study, participants include married individuals who are between the ages of 18 and 64 and identify as African American. The sample consisted of 102 African American participants, 56.9% males and 43.1% females. The average age of participants is 39. The average level of education completed is "some college." The average household income is between $35,000 and $39,000.

Dependent Variable

The dependent variable, marital satisfaction, was measured by participant's summed responses to 20 questions, items ranging from 1 (*Very Satisfied/Strongly Agree*) to 5 (*Very Dissatisfied/Strongly Disagree*). Sample questions include, "Taking all things together, how satisfied are you in your relationship with your spouse or partner?" "How satisfied are you with how well your spouse/partner listens to you?" and "My marriage/relationship hasn't gone quite as perfectly as I thought it might." The overall coefficient of reliability for the instrument is .941.

Independent Variables

The independent variables, work-family balance and work-family conflict, were measured by participant's responses to eight questions with regard to how individuals experience and perceive work-family balance and work-family conflict in their marriage. *Family-to-work conflict* was measured by the participant's response to six questions pertaining to components of work-family conflict such as how much conflict respondent faces in balancing work and family, how much conflict respondent's spouse faces in balancing work and family, respondent's family interferes with work, respondent's work interferes with family, spouse's family interferes with work, and spouse's work interferes with family. *Work-family balance* was measured by the participant's response to two questions pertaining to components of work-family balance such as respondent's perception of the fairness of the division of paid work and household labor and spouse's perception of the fairness of the division of paid work and household labor.

RESULTS

Work-Family Balance, Work-Family Conflict, and Marital Satisfaction among African Americans

A stepwise multiple regression analysis was conducted to estimate a model that best predicts levels of marital satisfaction among African Americans. The results of the stepwise analysis revealed that three of eight work-family factors emerged as significant predictors of marital satisfaction ($F = 12.29$; $p < .05$). With a beta of .230 ($p < .05$), the amount of conflict spouse face in balancing paid work and family life emerged as the strongest predictor of marital satisfaction, accounting for 16.6% of the variance in marital satisfaction. The second strongest factor was the amount of conflict the respondent faces in balancing paid work and family life ($\beta = .275$; $p < .05$) accounting for an additional 6.4% of the variance in marital satisfaction. The third strongest factor was work-family balance is unfair to the respondent ($\beta = .231$, $p < .05$) accounting for an additional 4.5% of the variance in marital satisfaction (Table 1).

These results indicate that higher levels of marital satisfaction are a function of lower amounts of conflict spouse faces in balancing paid work and family life, lower amounts of conflict respondent faces in balancing paid work and family, and the respondent not perceiving work-family balance as unfair to him- or herself. Overall, the model explains 27.5% of the variance in marital satisfaction

TABLE 1
Results of Multiple Regression Analysis—Predictors of Marital Satisfaction

Factor	R	$R2$	β	t	p	F	p
	.408	.166	.230	2.328	.022	19.735	.000
WFC faced by respondent	.480	.230	.275	3.017	.003	14.650	.000
WFB unfair to respondent	.525	.275	.231	2.460	.016	12.288	.000

($R = .525$). On the other hand, 72.5% of the variance in marital satisfaction is unaccounted for by this model.

$$\text{Marital Satisfaction} = 3.22 + (.07 \times \text{WFC faced by spouse})$$

$$+ (.09 \times \text{WFC faced by respondent}) + (.19 \times \text{WFB unfair to respondent})$$

Work-Family Balance, Work-Family Conflict, and Marital Satisfaction among African American Males

A stepwise multiple regression analysis was conducted to estimate a model that best predicts levels of marital satisfaction among African Americans males. The results of the stepwise analysis revealed that two of eight work-family factors emerged as significant predictors of marital satisfaction ($F = 8.44$; $p < .05$). With a beta of .315 ($p < .05$), the amount of conflict respondent faces in balancing paid work and family life emerged as the strongest predictor of marital satisfaction, accounting for 16.0% of the variance in marital satisfaction. The second strongest factor was the amount of conflict the respondent's spouse faces in balancing paid work and family life ($\beta = .292$; $p < .05$) accounting for an additional 7.8% of the variance in marital satisfaction (Table 2).

These results indicate that higher levels of marital satisfaction are a function of lower amounts of conflict respondent faces in balancing paid work and family life and lower amounts of conflict respondent spouses face in balancing paid work and family. Overall, the model explains 23.8% of the variance in marital satisfaction ($R = .488$). On the other hand, 76.2% of the variance in marital satisfaction is unaccounted for by this model.

$$\text{Marital Satisfaction} = 3.18 + (.10 \times \text{WFC faced by respondent}) + (.08 \times \text{WFC faced by spouse})$$

Work-Family Balance, Work-Family Conflict, and Marital Satisfaction among African American Females

A stepwise multiple regression analysis was conducted to estimate a model that best predicts levels of marital satisfaction among African Americans females. The results of the stepwise analysis revealed that one of eight work-family factors emerged as a significant predictor of

TABLE 2
Results of Multiple Regression Analysis—Predictors of African American Male Marital Satisfaction

Factor	R	$R2$	β	t	p	F	p
WFC faced by respondent	.408	.166	.230	2.328	.022	19.735	.000
WFC faced by spouse	.480	.230	.275	3.017	.003	14.650	.000

TABLE 3
Results of Multiple Regression Analysis—Predictors of African American Female Marital Satisfaction

Factor	R	R2	β	t	p	F	p
WFB fair to respondent and spouse	.504	.25.4	−.504	−3.78	.000	14.285	.000

marital satisfaction ($F = 14.29$; $p < .05$). With a beta of −.504 ($p < .05$), the respondent perceiving work-family balance as fair to both him or herself as well as his or her spouse emerged as the strongest predictor of marital satisfaction, accounting for 25.4% of the variance in marital satisfaction (Table 3).

These results indicate that higher levels of marital satisfaction are a function the respondent perceiving work-family balance as fair to herself as well as to her spouse. Overall, the model explains 25.4% of the variance in marital satisfaction ($R = .504$). On the other hand, 74.6% of the variance in marital satisfaction is unaccounted for by this model.

Marital Satisfaction = 3.84 + (−.345 × WFB is fair to respondent and respondent's spouse)

DISCUSSION

Impact of Work-Family Balance and Work-Family Conflict on African American Marital Satisfaction

This study revealed a negative relationship between African American marital satisfaction and work and family. Specifically, findings suggest the less conflict an individual and his or her spouse face in balancing paid work and family as well as the respondent not perceiving work-family balance as unfair to him or herself will result in higher levels of marital satisfaction. These findings are similar to previous studies (Barnett et al., 2003; Hammer & Thompson, 2003; Kossek & Ozeki, 1998) and indicate that similar to their European (Kossek & Ozeki, 1998) and Mexican American (Barnett et al., 2003) counterparts, African American levels of marital satisfaction are impacted in the same way by work-family balance and work-family conflict.

Also similar to findings by Barnett et al. (2003), whose study utilized a Mexican American sample, this study found that perceptions of work-family balance and work-family conflict are what most impacts marital satisfaction. Variables such as have you ever had to miss a family event due to work or vice versa did not significantly impact marital satisfaction. This may be due to the inevitable realization of individuals expecting to have to sometimes sacrifice one realm over the other, but their perception of how often they must sacrifice or how much conflict it causes is what impacts marital satisfaction.

This study also found that African American males' and females' level of marital satisfaction was a determinant of differing work-family conflict and work-family balance variables. African American women's level of marital satisfaction depends on wives' perception of work-family balance being fair to her as well as her spouse with the more fair a wife perceives work-family balance between her and her spouse, the more satisfied she is in her marriage. Males' level of marital satisfaction was determined by perception of work-family conflict to both him and his spouse. For African American males, higher levels of marital satisfaction are a function of lower amounts of conflict respondent faces in balancing paid work and family life and lower amounts of conflict respondent's spouse faces in balancing paid work and family. The difference between the wives' and husbands' levels of marital satisfaction is that wives' marital satisfaction depends on fairness of work-family balance while husbands' marital satisfaction depends on amount of work-family conflict felt by him and his wife.

What is interesting about the differences between husbands and wives in this case is that wives' main concern is fairness and views work and family from a work-family balance lens. As long as both husband and wife have obtained fairness in work-family balance, which is the enrichment obtained by engaging in both spheres, the more the wife is satisfied in her marriage. Husbands' marital satisfaction, on the other hand, depends on the level of conflict faced in balancing work and family. It is the work-family conflict lens that is utilized by African American husbands and best predicts their marital satisfaction. In other words, if work and family realms clash often, the less satisfied African American husbands will be in their marriage.

Implications for Social Workers

Work-family conflict and work-family balance affect African American marriages in the same way it affects their European and Mexican American counterparts. When work-family balance increases, marital satisfaction increases. When work-family conflict increases, marital satisfaction decreases. It is important for social workers working in marriage and family services or private practice to be aware of the impact of work and family challenges on marital satisfaction as well as be effectively trained in addressing these issues. Social work practitioners should routinely assess each client's work-family dynamics to determine their affect on marriage. Social work practitioners should be equipped with the knowledge and skills to help individuals, couples, and families increase work-family balance and decrease work-family conflict, which will in turn increase marital satisfaction. Strategies may include assisting clients in making adjustments to either their work realm, family realm, and/or spouses work realm and family realm. In addition, couples should consider soliciting available online services for competent child care so that they can create intimate time and activities for themselves.

This study revealed that different work-family variables contribute to husbands' verses wives' marital satisfaction. Husbands' marital satisfaction increases when work-family conflict is low. Wives' marital satisfaction increases when work-family balance is high and fair to both spouses. These differences indicate that social workers may need to discuss work-family challenges using different emphasis for husbands and wives. With wives, it might be important to emphasize work-family balance, ensuring wives that work and family can be compatible, complementary, and fair to both spouses. Social workers will need to help wives think of ways to increase work-family balance. When working with husbands, social workers may need to emphasize work-family conflict and help husbands strategize to find ways to decrease work-family conflict. When both spouses are present, social workers may need to help wives understand the husband's perspective using a work-family conflict lens and help husbands understand the wives perspective using a work-family balance lens.

Policy Implications

Social workers should actively engage in and advocate for policies that will increase work-family balance and decrease work-family conflict. Social workers can advocate for flexible hours, decreased work hours, and child care. Flexible hours would allow men and women the opportunity to work the hours required of them by their employer but during times that are more convenient for them. For example, if a parent has a child who needs to be to school by 8:00 in the morning, the parent should be allowed to adjust his or her schedule in order to take the child to school and then come to work shortly after as opposed to both parent and child having to be to work and/or school at the same time or parent having to be to work before the child. In addition, instead of the typical 40-hour-plus work week, policies should be considered that decrease the time spent at work, allowing individuals to spend more time with their families. Last, it is important that work-family policy prioritize child care. Jobs should be required to provide child care or a stipend that will afford parents the opportunity to seek child care if needed. This is especially crucial for parents working non-typical hours such as an overnight shift.

Future Research

In order to decrease work-family conflict and increase work-family balance, future research is required that examines the impact of current work-family policies; develops evidence-based practice aimed at reconciling work and family realms; and identifying additional factors that mediate the relationship between work and family. Examining the current impact of work-family policy, especially among African Americans, is important in understanding both the negative and positive effects of policy. If policy mandates a 40-plus-hour work week, this may have a negative effect on the family sphere because less time is designated to family. However, if policy mandates child care laws, this may have a positive impact for employees in both the work and family sphere by assisting parents in balancing work and family responsibilities.

Developing a track record of evidence-based practice aimed at reconciling work and family conflict is necessary in order to establish which programs and policies are effective and which are ineffective. It is not enough to shorten mandatory work hours from 40-plus a week to 35 hours a week if research shows that a 35-hour work week still has the same effect on work-family balance as a 40-plus-hour work week. Instead, mandatory work hours would need to be decreased to the point that research shows is making a positive impact on work and family life. Last, social scientists must identify variables that mediate the relationship between work and family and its impact on marital satisfaction. Protective factors should consistently be identified and implemented into both practice and policies in an effort to improve work-family balance thereby increasing marital satisfaction.

CONCLUSION

African American marital satisfaction is a function of work and family challenges. In order to increase marital satisfaction, social workers should assist clients in increasing work-family balance and decreasing work-family conflict as well as understand the differences in work-family variables that impact husbands' marital satisfaction compared to that of wives. Social workers must also advocate for work-family policies that will increase work-family balance and decrease work-family conflict, which will then increase marital satisfaction. The relationship between work-family conflict and marital satisfaction is important to family and community well-being as well as child outcomes. Social workers should strive to pay more attention to marriage work.

REFERENCES

Administration of Child and Families. (2006). *ACF Healthy Marriages, Initiative factsheet.* Washington, DC: Government Printing Office.

Amato, P. R., Booth, A. Johnson, D. R., & Rogers, S. J. (2003). Continuity and change in marital quality between 1980 and 2000. *Journal of Marriage and Family, 65,* 1–22.

Barnett, K. A., Del Campo, R. L., Del Campo, D. S., & Steiner, R. L. (2003). Work and family balance among dual-earner working-class Mexican-Americans: Implications for therapists. *Contemporary Family Therapy, 25*(4), 353–366.

Bianchi, S. M., & Milkie, M. A. (2010). Work and family research in the first decade of the 21st century. *Journal of Marriage and Family, 72,* 705–725.

Broman, C. L. (2005). Marital quality in black and white marriages. *Journal of Family Issues, 26,* 431.

Broman, C. L. (2002). Thinking of divorce, but staying married: The interplay of race and marital satisfaction. *Journal of Divorce and Remarriage, 37*(1/2), 151.

Broman, C. L. (1993). Race differences in marital well-being. *Journal of Marriage and Family, 55*(3), 724–732.

Bryant, C. M., Taylor, R. J., Lincoln, K. D., Chatters, L. M., & Jackson, J. S. (2008). Marital satisfaction among African Americans and Black Caribbeans: Findings from the National Survey of American Life. *Family Relations, 57,* 239–253.

Bulanda, J. R., & Brown, S. L. (2008). Working paper series 06-08: Race-ethnic differences in marital quality and divorce. Bowling Green, OH: Bowling Green State University, Center for Family Demographics Research.

Byron, K. (2005). A meta-analytic review of work-family conflict and its antecedents. *Journal of Vocational Behavior, 67,* 169–198.

Gareis, K. C., Barnett, R. C., Ertel, K. A., & Berkman, L. F. (2009). Work-family enrichment and conflict: Additive effects, buffering, or balance. *Journal of Marriage and Family, 71,* 696–707.

Greenhaus, J. H., & Beutell, N. J. (1985). Sources of conflict between work and family roles. *Academy of Management Review, 10,* 76–88.

Grzywacz, J. G., & Carlson, D. S. (2007). Conceptualizing work-family balance: Implications for practice and research. *Advances in Developing Human Resources, 9,* 455–471.

Hammer, L., & Thompson, C. (2003). Sloan work and family research network encyclopedia. Retrieved from http://wfnetwork.bc.edu/encyclopedia_entry.php?id=264

Hughes, E. L., & Parks, K. R. (2007). Work hours and well-being: The roles of work-time control and work-family interference. *Work & Stress, 21*(3), 264–278.

Kossek, E. E., & Ozeki, C. 1998. Work-family conflict, policies, and the job-life satisfaction relationship: A review and directions for organizational behavior/human resources research. *Journal of Applied Psychology, 83,* 139–149.

Lincoln, K. D., & Chae, D. H. (2010). Stress, marital satisfaction, and psychological distress among African Americans. *Journal of Family Issues, 31*(8), 1081–1105.

Loveless, S., & Holman, T. (2007). *The family in the new millennium: The place of family in human society.* Westport, CT: Praeger Publishers.

Mitchelson, J. K. (2009). Seeking the perfect balance: Perfectionism and work-family conflict. *Journal of Occupational and Organizational Psychology, 82,* 349–367.

Stone, E. A., & Shackelford, T. K. (2007). *Encyclopedia of social psychology.* Thousand Oaks, CA: Sage Publications.

Tatman, A. W., Hovestadt, A. J., Yelsma, P., Fenell, D. L., & Canfield, B. S. (2006). Work and family conflict: An often overlooked issues in couple and family therapy. *Contemporary Family Therapy, 28*(1), 39–51.

Teachman, J. D., Tedrow, L. M., and Crowder, K. D. (2000). The changing demography of America's families. *Journal of Marriage and the Family, 62,* 1234–1246.

Trent, K., & South, S. (2003). Spousal alternatives and marital relations. *Journal of Family Issues, 24,* 787–810.

U.S. Bureau of the Census. (2006). *Statistical abstract of the United States* (122nd ed.). Washington, DC: U.S. Government Printing Office.

Voyandoff, P. (2005). Toward a conceptualization of perceived work-family balance: A demands and resources approach. *Journal of Marriage and Family, 67,* 822–836.

Wilcox, W. B., Marquardt, E., Popnoe, D., & Whitehead, B. D. (2009). *State of our unions: Marriage in America 2009.* Charlottesville, VA: National Marriage Project and Institute for American Values.

Wong, S., & Goodwin, R. (2009). The impact of work on marriage in three cultures: A qualitative study. *Community, Work & Family, 12*(2), 213–232.

American Indian Perceptions of Paternal Responsibility

Gordon E. Limb and Jerilyn Tobler

School of Social Work, Brigham Young University, Provo, Utah, USA

Using data from the Fragile Families and Child Wellbeing Study, this study examined the issue of American Indian nonresident father rights and obligations. Findings revealed that both American Indian mothers and fathers supported visitation rights, but decision-making rights were not highly supported unless the father was paying child support. Both American Indian parents were similar in their views regarding paternal responsibilities. Therefore, while general father involvement intervention strategies may work for American Indians, it is important for practitioners to explore how American Indians define paternal involvement and to what extent they are willing to allow the nonresident father to participate in all aspects of the child's life.

In the United States, the number of children in single-mother families has increased at an alarming rate over the past four decades (Mather, 2010). Father absence has dramatically altered the dynamics of the family and continues to impact the role and expectations of fathers. In 2010, 34% of children under the age of 18 in the United States resided in homes operated by a single parent—most often a single mother (Annie E. Casey Foundation, 2010). While father absence is a concern generally, American Indian families are also experiencing an increase of single-parent households. For example, 52% of American Indian children lived in single-parent families in 2010 (Annie E. Casey Foundation, 2010).

Scholars have expressed concern that American Indian children living with a single parent are at greater risk than are children in the general population in a number of areas, often due to the complexity of hardships faced by American Indian families (Hummer & Hamilton, 2010; Sandefur & Liebler, 1997). Here, U.S. Census data show that American Indian children are less likely than many other racial/ethnic groups to reside with two parents, American Indian women are less likely to marry, and American Indians are more likely to face high unemployment and poverty rates (U.S. Census Bureau, 2011).

While a growing body of research exists that examines these issues generally, few studies have looked at the American Indian population. Using data from the Fragile Families and Child Wellbeing Study, this study adds to the previous research (see Lin and McLanahan, 2007) by examining American Indian mothers' and fathers' perspectives about nonresident fathers' financial support obligations, their rights to visit, and their rights to make decisions regarding the children with whom they do not live. The goal of this study is to provide awareness relating to American Indian parents and their perceptions of nonresident fathers' child support obligations and rights. Further, it is important to recognize differences in the context of cultural norms and expectations of American Indian parents and the promotion of positive relationships that impact the well-being of their children.

CHILD SUPPORT OBLIGATIONS

In the general population, the father's role traditionally has been viewed in terms of providing for his family economically (primary bread-winner) and socially (protection, discipline, moral guide, teacher, role model; Dudley & Stone, 2001; Lamb & Tamis-Lemonda, 2004; McLanahan & Beck, 2010). For American Indians, family roles are more interconnected, and the obligation to support economically and care for children has not traditionally been the sole expectation or responsibility of a father. Glover (2001) and Whitbeck (2006) both emphasize that the extended family, community, and tribe are viewed as collective pieces of the Native family circle and hold similar responsibilities and roles to the children as do a mother and father. Although their roles may be different, each system plays an important role in the well-being of the American Indian child.

Typically in the United States, the response to nonresident fathers' financial obligations has been to create strict child support regulations, stating that the general population perceives child support and visitation rights as interconnected (Lin & McLanahan, 2007). Here, the belief was that if the father paid child support, then he earned the right to visitation (Stewart, 2010), whereas if he did not keep up with his financial obligations, then his rights should be limited (Lin & McLanahan, 2007). Here, cultural considerations in the general population appear to be less important than the monetary aspect of his obligation. While many minority groups place importance on non-monetary aspects (e.g., connectedness, cohesion, support), regulations tend to focus on the monetary aspect over the cultural aspects.

Traditionally, when asked about default with child support payments, fathers listed unemployment issues, concerns that the mother was not spending child support money on children, and being denied access to their children as possible reasons (Klinman & Kohl, 1984). More recently, researchers found that the nonresident fathers' current marriage/relationship status and whether they have other biological children or step-children were also factors (Manning, Stewart, & Smock, 2003; Nepomnyaschy & Garfinkel, 2011).

Few studies have been conducted with American Indians to find out their specific views about child support obligations. What has been found is that people of color experience higher percentages of single-mother families, lower income levels, higher rates of poverty, and that cultural belief about gender and family are important factors to consider when determining paternal involvement (Hummer & Hamilton, 2010; Jackson, 1999). Although the ideal situation for American Indians is to have support from extended kin and community/tribe, many face great difficulty in being able to achieve it. The effects of poverty and unemployment on some reservations have led American Indians, including nonresident fathers, to move to urban areas where even greater difficulties are encountered, and the family can be left to cope without this support. White, Godfrey, and Moccasin (2006) note that "a loss of male influence in the American Indian life can be traced to a loss of cultural practices and traditions" (p. 50), and this has left many families in need of additional support. As a result, an examination of American Indian fathers' responsibilities and rights is warranted.

Father's Rights

Fatherhood has been identified as a *social role* for men and that the absence of this role has a negative impact on the well-being of children (Blackenhorn, 1995; Bzostek, 2008; Huang, 2006). American Indian fathers are traditionally expected to contribute great strength to the family system as teachers, guides, role models, and leaders (Glover, 2001; White et al., 2006). One study conducted on married Navajo Indian mothers/fathers found fathers to have a high involvement with their infant children (Hossain et al., 1999). This social role is a support that nonresident fathers can provide regardless of their financial circumstances, yet the standard approach has been on laws and policies that enforce financial obligations to their children instead of programs to encourage positive father-child relationships, thus leading to increased financial support (Curran, 2003).

Studies have found that mothers and children portray a desire to have the father involved in their life and to maintain a relationship with them (King & Heard, 1999; Laughlin, Farrie, & Fagan, 2009). In addition, Amato and Sobolewski (2004) found a trend of increased father involvement suggesting that fathers also wish to remain a part of their children's lives. For American Indians, the emotional aspects (connectedness, cohesion, support) of family are viewed as the most positive influence on child well-being (Teufel-Shone et al., 2005), suggesting that increased father involvement has many positive impacts. Thus scholars suggest that the stabilizing aspects of marriage serve more than just the function of the male/female union; it is an abiding, enduring, and necessary function of child well-being in Native culture (McLanahan, 2006).

Socio-Demographic Factors

When discussing individual positions held about nonresident fathers' economic and social responsibilities, a number of socio-demographic factors may influence attitudes and perceptions. For example, one study compared married and unmarried father's responses and found that the marital status of a father contributes to differences in views about paternal roles, with unmarried fathers less likely to strongly agree with statements about the father's role (McLanahan & Carlson, 2004). A father's socioeconomic status (especially education status) has been linked to an increase in likelihood that he will be involved with his children and provide financial support (Amato & Sobolewski, 2004; Conger, Conger, & Martin, 2010). Having other children, whether biological or step-children, can influence the level of involvement a nonresident father has with his children (Manning et al., 2003; Seltzer & Brandreth, 1994). Here, while blended families and step-children may not be the preferred family dynamic in American Indian culture, similar to the general population, it is not discouraged in cases such as domestic violence, substance abuse, abandonment, or irreconcilable differences (Net Industries, 2012). Scholars also suggest that a father's age or the timing he first enters into the fatherhood role impacts attitudes and levels of involvement with children (Cooney, Pedersen, Indelicato, & Palkovitz, 1993; Laughlin et al., 2009). Likewise, research has found that patterns and perceptions of father involvement vary significantly across racial or ethnic groups in the United States (Hummer & Hamilton, 2010; Sanderson & Thompson, 2002; Toth & Xu, 1999).

For American Indians, there are a number of socio-demographic impacts. As mentioned previously, American Indians were among the poorest groups in American society, with over 28% living in poverty (U.S. Census Bureau, 2011). American Indian parents were on average less educated when compared to the general population. Additionally, only about 22% of American Indians lived on reservations or tribal areas, meaning more and more Native families are living in urban areas and struggling with these unique challenges. This presents a unique challenge with regard to marriage and child rearing for these urban families. Some scholars suggest that the absence of urban American Indian fathers limits transference of important cultural knowledge, awareness, and appropriate male role models (e.g., being there) to the next generation (Shears, Bubar, & Hall, 2011; Urban Indian Health Institute, 2011), whereas in reservation areas, males in extended families can often fill in and provide this resource.

There is a gap in the literature when it comes to American Indian father research, particularly in the areas of nonresident father's rights and obligations. Therefore, the purpose of this study was to utilize Fragile Families data to examine urban American Indian mothers' and fathers' perspectives about nonresident fathers' financial support obligations, his rights to visit, and his rights to make decisions regarding the children with whom he does not live. As a result, this study sought to increase awareness of urban American Indian parents and their perceptions of nonresident fathers' obligations and rights.

METHOD

Data and Participants

This study uses data from the Fragile Families and Child Wellbeing study, a national, longitudinal study designed to examine the characteristics of unmarried parents, the relationships between them and the fathers, and the consequences for children (see Reichman, Teitler, Garfinkel, & McLanahan, 2001). The Fragile Families study follows a new birth cohort of approximately 4,900 children born between 1998 and 2000 (including 3,712 children born to unmarried parents and 1,186 children born to married parents) in 20 cities with populations over 200,000. The Fragile Families study uses a stratified random sampling design and, when weighted, the sample is representative of all births to unmarried parents in cities with populations over 200,000.

The Fragile Families study first interviewed mothers within 48 hours of birth while they were still in the hospital. Fathers were interviewed either in the hospital or wherever they could be located as soon as possible after the birth. Response rates for the baseline survey were 87% for unmarried mothers (82% for married mothers) and 75% for unmarried fathers (89% for married fathers). The total sample size includes 4,898 mothers and 3,830 fathers.

For the current study, data from the first wave of the Fragile Families study were examined, but the sample was restricted to only those mothers who self-identified as being American Indian. This yielded a total analysis sample of 222 mothers (comprising 4.5% of the total sample). Each mother's ID number was utilized to pair the fathers linked to them. After excluding 13 mothers and 61 fathers who did not answer all the survey questions regarding nonresident fathers' obligations and rights, the sample consists of 209 mothers and 161 fathers. Both fathers and mothers were asked survey questions related to their views about nonresident fathers' child support obligations and nonresident fathers' rights to visitation and decision making. Mothers' and fathers' individual socio-demographic information was controlled for in this study.

Independent Variables

Socio-Demographic Factors

For the current study, six socio-demographic variables were used to analyze opinions about nonresident fathers' obligations and rights: marital status (married versus unmarried), parenthood history (if have other children), education, socioeconomic status/household income, age, and gender.

The first measure, marital status, was dichotomous and asked respondents whether they were married to the baby's mother or father. The second measure, parenthood history, was also dichotomous and asked respondents, "Do you have other biological children?" A scale measure was used to determine mothers' and fathers' education level where respondents were asked about their "Highest grade of regular school that you completed" and recoded in into three categories: (1) Less Than High School (included no formal education, below the eighth grade, and some High School); (2) High School (included HS Diploma and GED); and (3) More Than High School (included some college, trade school, bachelor, or graduate degrees).

To determine mothers' and fathers' socioeconomic status, a scale measure was utilized and asked respondents what their total household income (before taxes) was for the last year and given the following choices (1) < 5,000, (2) 5 K–9,999, (3) 10 K–14,999, (4) 15 K–19,999, (5) 20 K–24,999, (6) 25 K–34,999, (7) 35 K–49,999, (8) 50 K–74,999, (9) > 75 K, and (10) No regular work. Other measures included a constructed father's and mothers' age variable for age at the time of the baby's birth. Gender was also utilized to compare male and female survey answers.

Dependent Variables

Child Support Obligations

Two dichotomous measures were used to determine views about nonresident fathers' child support obligations. For the first measure, respondents were asked, "If a mother has a new partner, do you think the baby's father should be required to provide financial support to his baby?" The second measure asked, "If the father has a new baby with another partner, do you think he should be required to provide support to his children from a previous relationship?"

Father's Rights

Two primary dichotomous measures were used to determine views regarding nonresident fathers' rights. The first measure focused on the fathers' right to visit the child. Respondents were asked whether they thought a nonresident father should have the right to see his child on a regular basis based on the following three items: (1) if the father provides financial support to the mother, (2) if the father cannot afford to provide financial support, and (3) if the father can afford to provide financial support but does not.

The second measure focused on the fathers' right to make decisions about how the child is raised. Respondents were asked whether they thought a nonresident father should have the right to make decisions about how the child is raised based on the following three items: (1) if the father provides financial support to the mother, (2) if the father cannot afford to provide financial support, and (3) if the father can afford to provide financial support but does not.

Data Analysis

The first set of analyses involved descriptive statistics to describe and compare the mothers' and fathers' opinions held about fathers' obligations and rights at the time of the child's birth. For these analyses, chi-square/Fisher's exact test were used to analyze differences between male and female answers. For the set of socio-demographic variables related to opinions about father obligations and rights, independent t tests and chi-square/Fisher's exact test were utilized to compare male and female answers.

The second set of analyses involved logistic regression models estimated to predict whether the identified six socio-demographic variables had a significant impact upon views held regarding nonresident fathers' obligations and rights. The models utilized in the regression analysis were the eight measures used for nonresident father's financial obligations and rights. The order of the eight models and what each one represented is listed as followed: (1) Father is obligated to pay if mother has a new partner; (2) father is obligated to pay if he has a new baby with another partner;

TABLE 1

American Indian Fathers' and Mothers' Perceptions Regarding Nonresident Fathers' Child Support Obligations and Rights

Fathers (N = 161)	%
1. Father is obligated to pay if mother has a new partner.	88.8*
2. Father is obligated to pay if he has a new baby with another partner.	97.5
3. Father has the right to see child if he pays.	97.5
4. Father has the right to make decisions about child if he pays.	90.7
5. Father has the right to see child if he is too poor to pay.	87.6
6. Father has the right to make decisions about child if he is too poor to pay.	73.9
7. Father has the right to see child if he can afford but does not pay.	28.0*
8. Father has the right to make decisions about child if he can afford but does not pay.	21.7

Mothers (N = 209)	
1. Father is obligated to pay if mother has a new partner.	83.7*
2. Father is obligated to pay if he has a new baby with another partner.	97.1
3. Father has the right to see child if he pays.	99.0
4. Father has the right to make decisions about child if he pays.	90.0
5. Father has the right to see child if he is too poor to pay.	88.0
6. Father has the right to make decisions about child if he is too poor to pay.	74.2
7. Father has the right to see child if he can afford but does not pay.	37.8*
8. Father has the right to make decisions about child if he can afford but does not pay.	25.4

*Significant difference ($p < .05$) between fathers and mothers on this measure.

(3) father has the right to see child if he pays; (4) father has the right to make decisions about child if he pays; (5) father has the right to see child if he is too poor to pay; (6) father has the right to make decisions about child if he is too poor to pay; (7) father has the right to see child if he can afford but doe not pay; and (8) father has the right to make decisions about child if he can afford but does not pay (Table 1). Each of the six socio-demographic variables was controlled for against the eight models in the regression analysis. In addition, a seventh demographic variable, father's race, was controlled for as the Fragile Families data included only 25.5% where the American Indian fathers' race matched the American Indian mothers' race. This suggests there is a strong multicultural influence in our American Indian sample.

RESULTS

Child Support Obligations

Table 1 contains the percentage of American Indian fathers and mothers who agreed with two statements regarding nonresident fathers' obligations. On the first measure, 85.9% of all respondents agreed that a father should be required to provide financial support to his baby, even if the mother had a new partner. Here, a significant difference was found between fathers and mothers in their perceptions of paternal obligation when the mother had a new partner. Whereas 88.8% of fathers agreed with this statement, mothers were less likely to agree that a nonresident father was obligated to pay child support when the mother had a new partner (83.7%).

With regard to the second measure, nearly all of the respondents (97.3%) considered a nonresident father obligated to provide child support to his previous children when he has a new baby with another partner. Although fathers and mothers did not differ significantly in their opinions on this measure, we found that mothers (97.1%) were slightly more likely to view that nonresident fathers did not have a financial obligation to pay child support in this situation (see Table 1), whereas slightly more fathers (97.5%) agreed that the obligation still existed for the nonresident father regardless of additional biological children.

Father's Rights

Table 1 also contains six measures that outline a nonresident father's rights to visit and make decisions about his child based on the following three conditions: if he paid child support, if he could not afford child support, and if he could afford to pay child support but did not. In general, both mothers and fathers were more likely to agree with nonresident fathers' rights to visitation than they agreed with his rights to make decisions.

On the first condition, regarding the birth father who provided child support, 98.4% of all respondents were in agreement that he has a right to visit the child, whereas 90.3% of mothers and fathers viewed that a paying birth father should have decision-making rights (see Table 1). The second condition asked about rights if the birth father was too poor to pay child support. When considering this scenario for the birth father, 87.8% of respondents supported visitation rights, and 74.1% supported decision making rights for him. The measures addressing the third condition, if the nonresident father could afford child support but did not pay it, resulted in the majority of respondents backing no rights to the child for a birth father in this circumstance. Only 32.9% of respondents agreed that the birth father should have visitation rights, and 23.5% agreed that he should have any decision-making power. A significant difference was found in fathers' and mothers' perceptions of father's rights to visit the child when the birth father could afford child support but did not. Here, mothers were more likely to agree with visitation rights.

Socio-Demographic Factors

Table 2 contains six socio-demographic factors comparing the birth fathers' and birth mothers' sample. Regarding parenthood history, 59.7% of respondents reported that they did have other biological children. No significant difference was found between genders, although mothers were more likely to have other biological children (60.8% compared to 58.4%).

The race and ethnicity factor ended up being more diverse than previously anticipated. Our hope was to have a matched sample of all American Indian fathers and mothers. We found that a total American Indian sample was not possible because only about one-fourth of American Indian mothers (25.5%) had their new baby with an American Indian father. The race with the highest percentage in our sample was those fathers who identified themselves as White (31.7%), the second highest being fathers who identified themselves as Hispanic/Other (31.1%), followed by Black (7.5%) and Asian (1.2%).

Another factor controlled for was that of fathers' and mothers' level of educational attainment. It was found that almost two-thirds (63.8%) of our sampled mothers and fathers had not completed a high school education (see Table 2). In addition, the smallest percentage of our respondents (17.3%) had achieved more than a high school education, which involved attending any college and/or completion of a technical trade school, bachelor, or graduate degree. No significant difference was found between genders, although mothers were more likely to have less than a high school education (67.9%) as compared to fathers (58.4%). It was also found that fathers were more likely to have gained a high school diploma or GED as compared to mothers.

Household income within the past year was found to be significantly different for fathers and mothers. The average income for fathers was higher (range of 10 K–1,999) than that of mothers (range of 5 K–9,999). It is also important to note that a high percentage (27.3%) of respondents

TABLE 2
American Indian Parents' Reports of Parental History and Other
Socio-Demographic Factors

Measures	Fathers % or M (SD)	Mothers % or M (SD)	χ^2 or t Test
Parental history			
Other biological children	58.4	60.8	
Marital status			
Married	26.1	20.6	
Unmarried	73.9	79.4	
Race/ethnicity			
White	31.7		
Black	7.5		
Hispanic/other	31.1		
American Indian	25.5	100	*
Asian	1.2		
Educational attainment			
More than high school	18.6	16.3	
High school	23.0	15.8	
Less than high school	58.4	67.9	
Household income	10 K–14,999	5 K–9,999	*
Age	26.9	24.5	*

*Significant difference ($p < .05$) between fathers and mothers on this measure.

answered that they did not know what their household income had been for the past year. With regard to age, a significant difference was found between mothers' average age (25 years old) and fathers' age (27 years old) at the time of the child's birth.

The last socio-demographic factor controlled for was that of fathers and mothers marital status. It was found that 77% of our respondents were unmarried at the time of the child's birth. No significant difference was found between genders in regard to marital status, but mothers were more likely to report being unmarried (79.4%) at the time of the birth as compared to fathers (73.9%).

In order to predict whether the identified six socio-demographic variables had significant impact upon views held regarding nonresident fathers' obligations and rights, a logistic regression was performed (see Table 3). Results of the regression showed that marital status had the most impact on fathers' and mothers' perceptions of nonresident fathers' obligations and rights. Marital status was found to be significant on five of the eight measures. Respondents' marital status was found most significant on measures asking whether a birth father who cannot afford to pay child support should see the child or whether he should have rights to make decisions about the child. If respondents were not married, they were more likely to disagree with these conditions.

Income was also found to be a significant factor among our respondents. The more income one had, the more likely they were to agree with nonresident father obligations to pay child support to previous children when he has a new baby and the more likely they were to disagree with nonresident father decision-making rights for a father who cannot afford child support. Age was found to be significant, with older individuals being more likely to disagree that a nonresident father should have rights to see the child when he can afford child support but does not pay (see Table 3). The more education one had, the more likely he was to agree with father's rights to decision making when he can afford support but does not and to agree with father's obligations to pay child support to child when mother has a new partner. Individuals who did not have other

TABLE 3
Nonresident Father Child Support Obligations and Rights Regressed against Respondents' Socio-Demographic Factors

Measures	(1) β (sig.β) Exp (β) p	(2) β (sig.β) Exp (β) p	(3) β (sig.β) Exp (β) p	(4) β (sig.β) Exp (β) p	(5) β (sig.β) Exp (β) p	(6) β (sig.β) Exp (β) p	(7) β (sig.β) Exp (β) p	(8) β (sig.β) Exp (β) p
Marital status	−.603 (.547) .094*	−1.103 (.332) .114	−1.101 (.333) .212	1.295 (3.650) .039**	1.317 (3.734) .017**	.835 (2.305) .012**	.295 (1.343) .280	.488 (1.629) .094**
Other biological children	.165 (1.179) .616	−.215 (.806) .772	−.143 (.867) .878	−.213 (.808) .570	−.205 (.815) .550	.164 (1.178) .524	.647 (1.910) .009***	.548 (1.730) .046**
Education	−.430 (.651) .080*	−.089 (.915) .853	.807 (2.240) .132	.275 (1.316) .233	.045 (1.046) .834	.028 (1.029) .863	−.212 (.809) .167	−.313 (.731) .057*
Income	−.081 (.922) .100	−.238 (.788) .037**	.132 (1.141) .346	.008 (1.008) .878	.078 (1.081) .122	.098 (1.103) .011**	−.011 (.989) .747	−.004 (.996) .912
Age	−.008 (.992) .777	.062 (1.064) .198	−.080 (.923) .418	−.015 (.985) .630	−.031 (.970) .308	−.013 (.987) .534	.050 (1.051) .022**	.035 (1.035) .144
Gender	−.355 (.701) .277	−.283 (.753) .682	.978 (2.659) .288	−.045 (.956) .902	.099 (1.104) .766	.020 (1.021) .935	.395 (1.484) .094*	.195 (1.215) .452

* $p < 0.10$. ** $p < 0.05$. *** $p < 0.01$.

biological children were more likely to disagree with a nonresident father's right to see his child and make decisions when he could afford support but did not pay.

Last, an important variable analyzed in this study was that of the father's race/ethnicity. Because we found our sample consisting of fathers from various ethnicities, we determined to explore whether race impacted the likelihood of fathers agreeing or disagreeing with measures related to nonresident father obligations and rights. While a logistic regression was conducted, and the father's race was controlled for, there was no significant difference found between a father's race and how he viewed nonresident father's obligations and rights.

DISCUSSION

Given that very little is known about the perceptions that American Indians have regarding paternal responsibility, the purpose of this study was to add critical information to the profession's knowledge base on this topic by examining American Indian mothers' and fathers' perspectives about nonresident fathers' obligations and rights. Results of this study point to three primary overall patterns. The first pattern indicated that there was generally no difference between perceptions held by American Indian parents and parents from the general population (see Lin & McLanahan, 2007). Here, we found that American Indian mothers and fathers were more likely to agree with rights to visitation than to agree with rights to decision making, which was similar to findings from studies that examined the entire Fragile Families sample. Embedded in this was the finding that marital status had the most impact on fathers' and mothers' perceptions of nonresident fathers' obligations and rights. This finding is similar to other studies that suggest marriage is an important stabilizing aspect in a relationship (McLanahan, 2006) and marital status having a positive impact on mothers perceptions of fathers obligation and rights (Lin & McLanahan, 2007).

The second pattern of results indicates that gender did not appear to have a significant impact on views. Our sampled mothers and fathers revealed comparable beliefs about obligations and rights, whereas, in previous research a more significant gender difference was found. For example, a Lin and McLanahan (2007) study revealed that mothers and fathers significantly differed on four measures regarding obligations and rights, but American Indian mothers and fathers differed on only two. Furthermore, we found gender to impact the expected likelihood of agreement on only one perception regarding visitation rights.

A third pattern emerged in controlling for socio-demographic factors. Overall, findings revealed that socio-demographics had an impact upon the way our sample perceived paternal responsibility. Of these, we found marital status to have the most significant impact. A consistent pattern appears with unmarried parents being more likely to disagree with nonresident fathers' decision-making rights. A large majority of our respondents were unmarried at the time of the new baby's birth. Studies have found that unmarried couples who cohabitate were much more likely to break up and be at a higher risk of their relationship ending in disruption (Bumpass & Hsien-Hen, 2000). In assuming that couples who are unmarried have a higher chance of separating, this would indicate that over three-fourths of these American Indian newborns are at risk of experiencing father absence in their life.

The overall pattern concerning child support obligations showed that mothers and fathers agreed that fathers should meet these obligations regardless of their nonresident status. This is consistent with other studies that reported the strongly held views regarding the traditional economic role of the father to support their offspring (see Dudley & Stone, 2001; Lamb & Tamis-Lemonda, 2004). Most American Indians in our study perceived a nonresident father as obligated to pay child support if he has a new baby with another partner. A smaller percentage agreed that a father was obligated to pay child support if the mother had a new partner. Here, the difference could be attributed to relationship status and/or step-children circumstances that have been shown in other studies to have an influence on perceptions (Manning et al., 2003).

When examining perceptions regarding nonresident fathers' rights, we found an overall pattern of his visitation rights being supported over his decision-making rights. The majority of American Indians support fathers being involved in their children's lives through visitation, but when it comes to making decisions about the child, very few agreed that nonresident fathers had the right to do this. This finding was consistent with previous studies that found mothers and children desire fathers to be involved, but the reality of this happening was shadowed by high levels of conflict in the relationship leading to dissatisfaction in father involvement (King & Heard, 1999; Laughlin et al., 2009).

In this study, we had the opportunity to compare not only mothers and fathers but fathers of various ethnicities. Based on previous research (e.g., Hummer & Hamilton, 2010; Sanderson & Thompson, 2002; Toth & Xu, 1999), race has been found to be a significant factor in perceptions related to paternal responsibility. Our study found, however, that overall, regardless of race or gender, individuals' perceptions of nonresident father obligations and rights do not differ significantly.

This study had several limitations. First, in trying to look specifically at American Indians we had a relatively small sample size with which to analyze. We also found the need to eliminate some respondents who did not answer each of the survey questions regarding nonresident father obligations and rights in order to run the analysis. Because of this small sample size, power to detect significant differences may have been more difficult. Second, because only a small proportion of American Indian mothers had children with American Indian fathers (roughly one-fourth), we were not able to obtain a full sample of American Indian respondents. With a larger sample, results may have been different if we included only American Indian mothers who had a child with an American Indian father. Third, this study used data from large urban areas. We foresee that findings may have been different if respondents were from rural or reservation areas. Taking the location and sample size factors into account, findings regarding American Indian perceptions about nonresident father obligations and rights may not be generalizable for all American Indians.

IMPLICATIONS

Recognizing the differences in the context of cultural norms and expectations suggests two implications for clinical practice with urban American Indians. First, because American Indian parents' views did not differ greatly from previous findings from the general Fragile Families population, it appears that intervention models and techniques that work for the general population might be effective for American Indians. These can include marriage and fatherhood programs (Cowan, Cowan, & Knox, 2010), group educational intervention programs (Doherty, Erickson, & LaRossa, 2006), and family group decision-making approaches (American Humane Association, 2010). While unique cultural elements must be considered with any intervention, practitioners can begin with models that have been found to be effective with the general population and then adapt them for an American Indian context.

Second, helping couples and families understand cultural norms and participate in traditional and cultural activities can aid in helping them stay connected and work together to promote positive relationships and outcomes. For American Indians in urban settings, helping them reconnect with extended family, traditional strengths, and urban Indian centers can also help father involvement. The Navajo Nation and organizations like the Denver Indian Family Resource Center and the Southern California Indian Center have developed curriculum and training programs that help urban Indian families and children reconnect with their cultural traditions. Here, it is important for clinicians to utilize appropriate urban resources and organizations into intervention strategies with American Indian fathers to give them a sense of identity, purpose, and responsibility. Doing this will not only benefit the father but improve his relationship with the mother and promote child well-being with the children.

CONCLUSION

Father absence is a concern that impacts all individuals and families, regardless of race or ethnicity. There is, however, an understanding of the need to involve fathers and how father involvement contributes to the well-being of children (Blackenhorn, 1995; Bzostek, 2008; Huang, 2006). The current study is an important step at beginning to address the issue of father absence for American Indians. This study found that American Indian parents support father involvement, as far as rights to visitation, but decision-making rights were not highly supported unless he was paying child support. Further, American Indian mothers and fathers were very similar in their views about paternal responsibilities, with marital status having the largest impact. Whereas American Indian parents' views did not differ greatly from the general population, one must still account for unique cultural expectations that may impact the way in which solutions to involve fathers should be handled in a clinical setting. In order to better advocate for the well-being of children, this study found that marital relationships in paternal responsibilities were important, and there continues to be a need to explore how American Indians define paternal involvement and to what extent they are willing to allow a nonresident father to participate in all aspects of a child's life.

REFERENCES

American Humane Association. (2010). Guidelines for family group decision making in child welfare. Retrieved from http://www.americanhumane.org/assets/pdfs/children/pc-fgdm-guidelinespdf.pdf

Amato, P. R., & Sobolewski, J. M. (2004). The effects of divorce on fathers and children: Nonresidential fathers and stepfathers. In M. E. Lamb (Ed.), *The role of the father in child development* (4th ed., pp. 341–368). Hoboken, NJ: John Wiley & Sons, Inc.

Annie E. Casey Foundation. (2010). Kids count data center. Retrieved from http://datacenter.kidscount.org/data/across states/Rankings.aspx?ind=107

Blackenhorn, D. (1995). *Fatherless America: Confronting our most urgent social problem.* New York, NY: Harper.

Bumpass, L. L., & Hsien-Hen, L. (2000). Trends in cohabitation and implications for children's family contexts in the United States. *Population Studies, 54*(1), 29–41.

Bzostek, S. H. (2008). Social fathers and child well-being. *Journal of Marriage and Family, 70*(4), 950–961.

Conger, R. A., Conger, K. J., & Martin, M. J. (2010). Socioeconomic status, family processes, and individual development. *Journal of Marriage and Family, 72*(3), 685–704.

Cooney, T. M., Pedersen, F. A., Indelicato, S., & Palkovitz, R. (1993). Timing of fatherhood: Is "on time" optimal? *Journal of Marriage and the Family, 55*(1), 205–215.

Cowan, P. A., Cowan, C. P., & Knox, V. (2010). Marriage and fatherhood programs. *Future of Children, 20*(2), 205–230.

Curran, L. (2003). Social work and fathers: Child support and fathering programs. *Social Work, 48*(2), 219–227.

Doherty, W. J., Erickson, M. F., & LaRossa, R. (2006). An intervention to increase father involvement and skills with infants during the transition to parenthood. *Journal of Family Psychology, 20*(3), 438–447.

Dudley, J. R., & Stone, G. (2001). *Fathering at risk: Helping nonresidential fathers.* New York, NY: Springer Publishing.

Glover, G. (2001). Parenting in Native American families. In N. B. Webb (Ed.), *Culturally diverse parent-child and family relationships: A guide for social workers and other practitioners* (pp. 205–231). New York, NY: Columbia University Press.

Hossain, Z., Chew, B., Swilling, S., Brown, S., Michaelis, M., & Philips, S. (1999). Fathers' participation in childcare within Navajo Indian families. *Early Child Development and Care, 154*, 63–74.

Huang, C. C. (2006). Child support enforcement and father involvement for children in never-married mother families. *Fathering, 4*(1), 97–111.

Hummer, R. A., & Hamilton, E. R. (2010). Race and ethnicity in fragile families. *Future of Children, 20*(2), 113–131.

Jackson, A. (1999). The effects of nonresident father involvement on single black mothers and their young children. *Social Work, 44*(2), 156–166.

King, V., & Heard, H. E. (1999). Nonresident father visitation, parental conflict, and mother's satisfaction: What's best for child's well-being? *Journal of Marriage and the Family, 61*(2), 385–396.

Klinman, D. G., & Kohl, R. (1984). *Fatherhood U.S.A. The first national guide to programs, services, and resources for and about fathers.* New York, NY: Garland Publishing.

Lamb, M. E., & Tamis-Lemonda, C. S. (2004). The role of the father: An introduction. In M. E. Lamb (Ed.), *The role of the father in child development* (4th ed., pp. 1–31). Hoboken, NJ: John Wiley & Sons, Inc.

Laughlin, L., Farrie, D., & Fagan, J. (2009). Father involvement with children following marital and non-marital separations. *Fathering: A Journal of Theory, Research, & Practice about Men as Fathers, 7*(3), 226–248

Lin, I. F., & McLanahan, S. S. (2007). Parental beliefs about nonresident fathers' obligations and rights. *Journal of Marriage and the Family, 69*(2), 382–398.

Manning, W. D., Stewart, S. D., & Smock, P. J. (2003). The complexity of fathers' parenting responsibilities and involvement with nonresident children. *Journal of Family Issues, 24*(5), 645–667.

Mather, M. (2010, May). *U.S. children in single-mother families.* Data brief. Washington DC: Population Reference Bureau.

McLanahan, S. S. (2006). Fragile families and the marriage agenda. In L. Kowaleski-Jones & N. H. Wolfinger (Eds.), *Fragile families and the marriage agenda* (pp. 1–21). New York, NY: Springer.

McLanahan, S., & Beck, A. N. (2010). Parental relationships in fragile families. *Future of Children, 20*(1), 17–37.

McLanahan, S. S., & Carlson, M. S. (2004). Fathers in fragile families. In M. E. Lamb (Ed.), *The role of the father in child development* (4th ed., pp. 368–397). Hoboken, NJ: John Wiley & Sons, Inc.

Nepomnyaschy, L., & Garfinkel, I. (2011). Fathers' involvement with their nonresident children and material hardship. *Social Service Review, 85*(1), 3–38.

Net Industries. (2012). American Indian families-American Indian child welfare. Retrieved from http://family.jrank.org/pages/76/American-Indian-Families-American-Indian-Child-Welfare.html

Reichman, N. E., Teitler, J. O., Garfinkel, I., & McLanahan, S. S. (2001). Fragile families: Sample and design. *Children and Youth Services Review, 23*, 303–326.

Sandefur, G. D., & Liebler, C. A. (1997). The demography of American Indian families. *Population Research and Policy Review, 16*, 95–114.

Sanderson, S., & Thompson, V. L. S. (2002). Factors associated with perceived paternal involvement in childrearing. *Sex Roles, 46*(3–4), 99–111.

Seltzer, J. A., & Brandreth, Y. (1994). What fathers say about involvement with children after separation. *Journal of Family Issues, 15*(1), 49–77.

Shears, J., Bubar, R., & Hall, R. C. (2011). Understanding fathering among urban Native American men. *Advances in Social Work, 12*(2), 201–217.

Stewart, S. D. (2010). Children with nonresident parents: Living arrangements, visitation, and child support. *Journal of Marriage and Family, 72*(5), 1078–1091.

Teufel-Shone, N. I., Staten, L., Irwin, S., Rawiel, U., Bravo, A. B., & Waykayuta, S. (2005). Family cohesion and conflict in an American Indian community. *American Journal of Health Behavior, 29*, 413–422.

Toth, J. F., & Xu, X. (1999). Ethnic and cultural diversity in fathers' involvement: A racial/ethnic comparison of African American, Hispanic, and White fathers. *Youth and Society, 31*(1), 76–99.

Urban Indian Health Institute. (2011). Discussions with urban American Indian and Alaska Native parents: Keeping babies healthy and safe. Retrieved from http://www.uihi.org/wp-content/uploads/2011/05/Discussions-with-Urban-American-Indian-and-Alaska-Native-Parents.pdf

U.S. Census Bureau. (2011). American Indian and Alaska Native heritage month: November 2011. Retrieved from http://www.census.gov/newsroom/releases/archives/facts_for_features_special_editions/cb11-ff22.html

Whitbeck, L. B. (2006). Some guiding assumptions and a theoretical model for developing culturally specific preventions with Native American people. *Journal of Community Psychology, 34*(2), 183–192.

White, J. M., Godfrey, J., & Moccasin, B. I. (2006). American Indian fathering in the Dakota Nation: Use of Akicita as a fatherhood standard. *Fathering, 4*(1), 49–69.

Single Parenting in the African American Community: Implications for Public Policy and Practice

Ingrid Phillips Whitaker

Department of Sociology and Criminal Justice, Old Dominion University, Norfolk, Virginia, USA

Mark M. Whitaker and Kanata Jackson

Department of Management, School of Business, Hampton University, Hampton, Virginia, USA

The percentage of female-headed African American families has increased significantly since the 1960s. It is now estimated that over half of all African American children will grow up in a female-headed household. This article examines factors related to the formation of these households as well as the challenges associated with these households. Policies and programs that have been implemented to treat these families are examined.

INTRODUCTION

In 1965, Daniel Patrick Moynihan ignited a firestorm with the publication of *The Negro Family: A Case for National Action*. In his publication, Moynihan drew attention to the growth of single-parent families (particularly female-headed households) in the African American community (Moynihan, 1965). Moynihan thrust into the public arena not only a segment of the population that was growing in size but also a population that was diverging from what he viewed as mainstream America. The report also drew attention to the problems created by this population. Among other things, Moynihan argued these families would be responsible for intergenerational poverty, low educational attainment of children, and ultimately, the creation of intergenerational single-parent households. When Moynihan's report was published in 1965, approximately 25% of African American Families were headed by single women. By 2010, that percentage has risen to 47%. It is now estimated that nearly 70% of all African American children are born to mothers who are not married (McLanahan, Haskins, Garfinkel, Mincy, & Donahue, 2010).

The issue of single parenting in the African American community has historically been framed as a social problem in the literature on families as well as public policy literature. The framing of this issue as a social problem has primarily focused on women who have never been married and have children out of wedlock. Families that are single-parent households due to divorce or the death of a spouse have not been framed as a social problem in the literature. The examination of single-female–headed households that are formed due to out-of-wedlock births has focused on the problems associated with these households. Typically, studies of these families have drawn attention to the factors that lead to the creation of these families. These factors have included: shortages of men, unemployment of men, high divorce and separation rates, and cultural attitudes that condone out-of-wedlock childbearing. In addition, the economic problems associated with these families have also been examined. In particular, the feminization of poverty and reliance on welfare are two salient economic issues related to single-parent female-headed households. Finally, the question of whether children growing up in these families experience compromised well-being outcomes has also been examined.

The problems that have historically been identified with single-parent families have informed public policies that have been designed to treat these families. Public policies related to these families have focused on three areas that usually seek to address these problems through a patriarchal approach. Public policies designed to treat single-female–headed households have included (1) the replacement of absent fathers through income maintenance programs (such as the Mothers Pensions programs, AFDC and then TANF); (2) the making of mothers into both caretaker and bread winner (through welfare reform initiatives); and more recently, and (3) an emphasis on marriage initiatives for poor women. What has typically been marginalized when it comes to policy has been an emphasis on approaches that focus on helping to strengthen these families as single-parent families and strengthening resources in communities that do not just reach these families but all families. This alternative approach would require incorporating a much stronger ecological perspective in the analysis of the problems facing single-female–headed families and the implementation of more universal programs rather than categorical means tested programs. Many have argued that such an approach would be more acceptable in the public's view, and consequently, would garner more support for funding compared to programs that specifically target a particular stigmatized portion of the population.

This paper will examine why African American single-female–headed households are viewed as a problem, how public policy has approached the issue of single-female–headed households in the African American community, and present alternative approaches to the dominant public policy framework that has not garnered as much attention but may hold promise in providing these families with the support they need.

In particular, African American female-headed families have also been examined from a strengths perspective. The strengths perspective emphasizes the adaptive nature of African American families. Within this framework, female-headed households are touted as a family form that has increased in the African American community in response to structural factors that have limited the availability of marriage partners as well as the durability of marriages in the African American community (Billingsley, 1968, 1992; Foster, 1983; Littlejohn-Baker & Darling, 1993; Hill, 2003). This perspective also draws attention to the unique cultural attributes of African American families, such as the prevalence of extended kinship family structure. In many instances, extended kin may offer African American female-headed families the instrumental, emotional, and parenting support that is needed in the absence of a male partner in the home (Foster, 1983). While this particular framework has been applied to the examination of female-headed households, it has received marginal attention in the public policy discourse concerning these families.

Embedded in this strengths perspective is the examination of how the extended kinship network enhances the instrumental and expressive resources of African American families (Littlejohn-Blake & Darling, 1993). Historically, the dominant framework used to examine female-headed families in the African American community has been one that uses White nuclear families as the yardstick for comparison. This perspective fails to take into account that all African family structures are far more likely to be extended compared to their White counterparts. Subsequently, African American female-headed families are far more likely to have access to instrumental and emotional sources of support that extend beyond themselves and immediate family.

PROBLEMS ASSOCIATED WITH SINGLE-FEMALE–HEADED HOUSEHOLDS IN THE AFRICAN AMERICAN COMMUNITY: A VIEW FROM THE LITERATURE

The Creation of Single-Female–Headed Households in the African American Community

Decades after the publication of Moynihan's report, research on single-female–headed families has tried to answer the question why African American families have such a high incidence of female headship. The research on this issue has placed emphasis on a number of factors: the limited number of available and acceptable marriage partners for African American women, higher separation and divorce rates for African American married couples, and shifts in attitudes toward marriage and childbearing in the African American community.

One of the most popular explanations concerning the higher rates of female-headed households in the African American community is the limited availability of African American males who are considered potential marriage partners (Wilson, 1987, 1996). Given the limited availability of "desirable" men of marrying age, some researchers have argued that never-married women of childbearing age in the African American community have contributed to the higher incidence of female-headed households in this community. Researchers who adhere to the male marriage pool argument cite factors not necessarily related to a conscious/deliberate choice of women to have children out of wedlock but the limited availability of men to form stable desirable partnerships with (Wilson, 1987, 1996).

The limited availability of African American men compared to African American women of marrying age has been attributed to a number of factors, including but not limited to, changes in the labor market and employment rates for African American males, incarceration rates for African American men, and morbidity and mortality rates in this population (Wilson, 1987, 1996; Rolison, 1992; Baker, 1999).

Employment

With respect to employment, Wilson (1987) has argued that after WWII, African American men experienced a decline in their employability because of shifts that have occurred in the structure of the American labor market and the continued limited educational attainment for African American men. Specifically, Wilson sites the decline in manufacturing and production jobs in inner cities. These jobs according to Wilson have been largely replaced by service sector jobs which offer low pay and limited benefits. These changes have created Black male underemployment and high levels of unemployment. These two factors are associated with an increase in single-female–headed households (Rolison, 1992; Baker, 1999). The relationship between the increase in single-female–headed households and Black male underemployment and unemployment is a reflection of factors men and women consider before making the decision to marry. One of the most salient factors in this consideration is the economic stability of the marriage partners, particularly the men. Black women do not diverge from this ideological foundation. Black women tend not to marry or remain in marriages when they feel the costs of marriage are greater than the potential benefits they will reap from the marriage (Staples, 1985).

This pattern is partially attributed to the nature of labor force participation for African American women. In particular, African American women have had higher rates of labor force participation compared to their White counterparts. This is especially true after WWII. African American women have experienced a smaller income difference compared to their White counterparts (Ricketts 1989). Thus African American women have historically had less to gain from marriage (at least economically) compared to their White counterparts.

Incarceration

Since the 1970s, there has been a boom in the prison population in the United States. In 1975, 100 per 100,00 of the resident population was incarcerated. By 2001, the number had risen to 472,000 per 100,000 residents (Pettit & Western, 2004). What has been particularly disturbing about this growth is the disproportionate percentage of African American men who are represented in the prison population.

African American men represent a disproportionate percentage of the prison population in the United States (Pettit & Western, 2004; Western & Pettit, 2000; Roberts, 2004; Unnever, 2008). According to Roberts, "Most of the people sentenced to time in prison today are black." For African American men born between 1965 and 1969, 20% had served time by their early thirties. In addition, within this same cohort, 30% of those without a college education and 60% of high school drop-outs were in prison by 1999 (Pettit & Western, 2004). By the end of 2002, of the approximately 2 million persons who were imprisoned in the United States, 586,700 were Black. African Americans are eight times more likely to spend time in prison compared to their White counterparts (Roberts, 2004). African American men face a 28.5% risk of entering prison compared to their White counterparts, who face a 4.4% risk (Pettit & Western, 2004). These statistics are particularly problematic given the age range at which African American men are entering prison at the highest rate. A significant portion of the population entering prison is of marriage age. Thus, the disproportionate rate of incarceration for African American males has also contributed to a limited marriage pool for African American women in that incarceration simply removes potential marriage partners from the community. However, there is also evidence that incarceration diminishes the economic prospects of men in the future (which is tied to women's decision to marry) and may cultivate antisocial behaviors tat prevent men from forming stable relationships with women (Lopoo & Western, 2005).

One of the consequences of incarceration is what is termed invisible punishment (Travis, 2002). Invisible punishment refers to the laws and practices that have the effect of excluding those that have been incarcerated from full civic and economic participation upon release from prison. In particular, having a criminal record excludes participation in certain professions (Travis, 2002; Roberts, 2004). This limits the number of potential employment opportunities for African American men. In addition, even when jobs allow for the employment of those who have a criminal record, the stigmatization associated with being incarcerated is difficult to overcome. Employers are reluctant to hire men, especially African American men, who have been incarcerated.

Attitudes toward Marriage and Childbearing

Another factor that has been examined with respect to the formation of these households in the African American community is shifting attitudes toward marriage and childbearing among women in general that may also be shared by African American women. Researchers have demonstrated that shifts in attitudes toward marriage and childbearing have occurred across racial and ethnic groups in the United States (Akerlof, Yellen, & Katz, 1996). Women are either delaying marriage or not marrying at all. In addition, it has become more acceptable to have children out of wedlock. However, within the African American community, the decision to not marry or delay marriage may be only partially related to shifting attitudes concerning marriage among African American women. Some research suggests that African American women still hold very traditional attitudes about marriage (Chaney, 2011; King, 1999). In addition to holding rather traditional views about marriage, for African American women, motherhood is a defining characteristic of womanhood (Chaney, 2011). Thus, even though African American women may have higher rates of non-marriage the fact that they have a high percentage of out-of-wedlock births may be more associated with the limited availability of men rather than drastic shifts in attitudes toward marriage within this population. Out-of-wedlock childbearing may partially be a reflection of the importance African American women place on childbearing even though marriage may not be an option.

Morbidity and Mortality among African American Men

Finally, there has been some attention given to the extent to which the higher morbidity and lower life expectancy rates for African American men have also contributed to their removal from the marriage pool. African American men experience higher death rates compared to their White counterparts due to heart disease, cancer, homicide, and HIV infection (Rich, 2000). African American men lag behind White males in life expectancy by 7.1 years (Rich, 2000). In addition, African American men are at higher risk for preventable diseases. The shorter life expectancy of African American men is clearly a factor that removes them from the marriage pool. However, the morbidity rates associated with African American men removes some of them from the marriage pool indirectly. Health and mental health issues that prevent participation in the labor market contribute to the limited participation or non-participation of African American men in the labor market, thus making them less acceptable as marriage partners.

The nature of health care in the United States has contributed to the morbidity rates for African American men. In particular, the provisions of health care in the country has historically been linked to access to health insurance. Access to health insurance has been derived from two paths in the United States: employment and social welfare. The availability of health insurance through employment for African American men has been limited by the high rates of unemployment experienced by this population even in non-recessionary times as well as the disproportionate representation of African American men in jobs that offer no health insurance benefits. While private health insurance through employment is limited for African American men, access to Medicare and Medicaid (the two major social welfare health insurance programs) is also limited. African American men have a much shorter life expectancy compared to their White male counterparts and African American women. Consequently, a lower proportion of African American men are insured by Medicare because of their shorter life expectancy. Coverage under Medicare does not begin until the age of 65. In addition, since Medicare is premised on paying a health insurance tax through employment, a disproportionate percentage of African American men do not qualify for the benefit based on the type of work they may have engaged in during the course of their lives. While Medicaid is an alternative form of coverage for medical care, the program is a public assistance program, and eligibility for the program has increasingly become the responsibility of individual states. African American men who work may not meet the eligibility guidelines for Medicaid based on their earnings.

Marriage Dissolution

Finally, while the divorce rate across racial and ethnic groups has increased and remains high in the United States, the divorce and separation rate for African American married couples has been particularly high. (Goodwin, 2003). While 32% of European American marriages end in divorce within the first 10 years, 47% of African American marriages end in divorce within the same time period (Goodwin, 2003). Thus, a portion of the increase in single-female–headed households is due to marriage dissolution rather than women who have never been married.

A number of explanations have been posited for the high divorce rates among African American couples. Most of these explanations focus on structural factors and conditions, relationship issues that are particularly unique to African American couples, and the convergence of these issues in producing strains in African American marriages. The structural explanations that have been put forth to explain the higher rates of marriage dissolution for African American couples include the employment differential between African American men and women as well as the imbalance in the gender ratio between African American men and women (Dickson, 1993; Pinderhughes, 2002). It has been noted that for the past few decades, the number of employed African American women has exceeded the number of employed African American men (Holzer, 2009). This employment imbalance between African American men and women has been linked to the declining availability of jobs that traditionally employed African American men (namely manufacturing jobs). In addition to the employment imbalance, African American men and women are also faced with a gender ratio imbalance (Dickson, 1993; Pinderhughes, 2002). Black women continue to outnumber Black men demographically. However, the imbalance in the gender ratio is further exacerbated by factors that take African American men, who are available, out of the marriage pool. These factors include unemployment, drug use and drug addiction, and incarceration.

The above-mentioned structural factors are related to many of the relational factors that lead to much higher marriage dissolution for African American couples. First, the imbalance in the gender ratio between African American men and women suggests that because of the shortage of available men, they are at an advantage in the marriage relationship. African American men may not have to work as hard to maintain relationships or may even decide not to completely commit to a relationship (Dickson, 1993). This gender ratio imbalance also has implications for how women view marriage. Women grow up with a message of self-reliance. Consequently, the self-reliance that is fostered in African American women may lead them to view marriage as more expendable (Dickson, 1993).

In addition to the strains in marriage discussed above, research has also pointed to the issue of the perception of manhood for African American men. In particular, the expectation of fulfilling the provider role for African American men may cause strain in marriages for two reasons. First, African American men are more likely to experience unemployment and underemployment during the course of their lifetime. In addition, given the educational and occupational attainment of African American women, it is likely that women may out-earn their spouses during the course of their marriage. These economic issues may place strain on marriages and lead to marriage dissolution (Pinderhughes, 2002). Coupled with strains created concerning issues related to the provider role are strains created by the invisibility and lack of power African American men may experience in the larger society. African American men may seek to have more power in the home to compensate for their perception of having limited power outside the home (Penderhughes, 2002). This expectation of having more power in the home may create conflicts in marriages given the level of independence and self-sufficiency that is fostered in African American women.

POVERTY AND WELFARE DEPENDENCY AMONG SINGLE-FEMALE–HEADED HOUSEHOLDS IN THE AFRICAN AMERICAN COMMUNITY

Two issues that have garnered a great deal of attention with respect to single-female–headed families in the African American community are the level of poverty these families experience and the extent to which these families are likely to rely on welfare support.

Feminization of Poverty among African American Female-Headed Households

The feminization of poverty has a relatively long history in the literature on women and their economic well-being. Women are more likely to experience poverty at some point in their lives compared to their male counterparts. According to the 2010 Census, approximately 15% of the U. S. population was considered officially poor. The percentage of men who were considered poor that year was 21.7% compared to 24.1% of women (DeNavas-Walt, Proctor, & Smith, 2011). The feminization of poverty literature also demonstrates that single women who are heads of households tend to have much higher rates of poverty compared to their married counterparts or even single men who are heads of households. According to the 2010 Census, 6.2% of married-couple families were below the poverty line in the United States compared to 31.6% of female-headed households. Men who were heads of household had a poverty rate of 15.8% for the same Census year. In addition, being a racial minority tends to increase the chances of experiencing poverty for single-female–headed households. According to the 2010 Census, 41% of Black female-headed families were poor in 2010 (DeNavas-Walt et al., 2011). It has also been noted that African American single-female–headed families are more likely to live in areas with much higher concentrations of poverty compared to their white counterparts. Thus, these families are more likely to experience the isolating effects associated with being poor (McClanahan & Garfinkel, 1989).

Since African American women who are single heads of households experience a much higher rate of poverty compared to their White counterparts, it has also been noted that African American children are far more likely to experience poverty at some point in their lifetimes. According to the U.S. Census of 2010, 22% of all persons under the age of 18 were considered poor in the United States. For Black children, 39.1% were considered poor (DeNavas-Walt et al., 2011). Despite the limited economic resources African American female-headed households experience, there is evidence that these households have access to social support networks that in many instances enhances the stability and survivability of these households (Dominguez & Watkins, 2003; Jayakody & Kalil, 2002; McCreary & Dancy, 2004; Harknett & Hartnett, 2011; Persaud, Gray, & Hunt, 1999).

African American female-headed households that were living in poverty reported using what they considered to be family members (blood and non-blood members) as well as friends who spanned across generations and households for a number of purposes. These included providing child care, financial support, emotional support, and companionship (McCreary & Dancy, 2004). While social support networks are used by women primarily for survival needs, Dominguez and Watkins (2003) argue that single-female–headed households also use what they refer to as social leverage networks. These are networks that provide information and other types of resources that lead to socioeconomic mobility. One of the major sources of mobility for these women are the connections they form in the work place (Dominguez & Watkins, 2003). Bridges to opportunities were acquired by women through the connections they had with co-workers and or supervisors. Thus, employment plays a major role in women accessing diverse opportunities that they might otherwise not have access to in their more insular support networks. Of particular interest for many of these households is the presence of social fathers in these families. Social fathers are men such as brothers, uncles, grandfathers, and friends who play a significant role in the stability of the home and the positive development of children (Jayakody & Kalil, 2002). Social fathers were especially important to women in offering them financial support and providing a male role model in the household.

Finally, there is evidence that religion also plays a significant role in single mothers successfully raising children to succeed (Persaud et al., 1999). Children of single mothers reported their mothers' belief in a supreme being playing a significant role in their success. The ability of single African American women to exhibit resiliency in difficult times is partially linked to spirituality and church involvement. According to Brodsky (1999), single African American mothers not only viewed involvement in church as a form of instrumental support but also a source of guidance and inspiration that was obtained from various members of the church.

Welfare Dependency

The prevalence of economic insecurity among African American female-headed households increases the chances of these households relying on public assistance for support. Subsequently, African American female-headed households are disproportionately represented among the population receiving TANF benefits. For example, in 2009, the percentage of married couple families receiving TANF benefits in some of the last 12 months was 1.4% compared to 4% of single-male-headed families and 12.5% of single-female–headed families (Irving, 2011). In examining the population of TANF recipients in the United States, 66.3% of TANF families were single-female–headed families compared to 27.6% that were headed by married couples and 6.1% headed by men only (Irving, 2011). The issue of female-headed and Black families being disproportionately represented on the TANF and formerly on AFDC has been an issue of contention for decades. The major policy concern with what many perceive as welfare dependency is the disproportionate percentage of African American female-headed households that rely on public assistance support and, until the passage of the Personal Responsibility Work Opportunity Reconciliation Act (PRWORA) of 1996, the perception that these women spent too much time on welfare rather than working. What has not been largely discussed is the extent to which the PRWORA, while trying to promote marriage, family stability, and self-sufficiency, in actuality created additional strains in male-female relationships and in many instances promoted further economic instability for these families.

Under TANF, women are required to provide information on the identity of the father or fathers of their children. The rationale for this type of disclosure is that unlike its predecessor AFDC, TANF is considered a temporary form of child support that provides for the care of children until the non-custodial parent can provide that support through Child Support Enforcement. In states that have adapted particularly strong Child Support Enforcement Policies in conjunction with TANF, unmarried couples are likely to experience more conflict that results in reducing union formation through marriage (Carlson, Garfinkel, McLanahan, Mincy, & Primus, 2004). In particular, fathers who are allowed to contribute to the mother of their child or children informally (rather than through child support enforcement) are more likely to have favorable relationships with the mother of their children. These fathers do not have to endure the pressures associated with formally being committed to pay child support. In addition, these arrangements are more likely to result in men and women seeing themselves as sharing resources for the care of their children, thus fostering more positive attitudes toward one another (Carlson et al., 2004).

Social Well-Being Outcomes for Children Growing Up in Single-Female–Headed Households in the African American Community

Given the limited economic resources available to a disproportionate percentage of female-headed households, some of the research on these households has called into question whether the children raised in these households experience a compromised quality of life and well-being compared to children raised in two-parent-headed households. The issue of the well-being of children raised in single-female–headed households is often linked to two issues. First, researchers have examined the extent to which the economic distress associated with these families is associated with poor outcomes for children. Second, researchers have also examined the extent to which a one-parent family may not afford children the same resources in time commitment that two-parent families may afford children. Researchers have examined factors such as educational achievement, behavioral problems, as well as mental health outcomes.

The Fragile Families and Child Well Being Study out of Princeton and the Brookings Institute have examined the plight of children raised in two-parent and single-parent households. The research from comprehensive study indicates that a number of demographic, human capital, health, and household stability characteristics of single-parent families are related to the outcomes children experience in these families. In particular, the findings indicate that women who are single heads of household tend to be younger than their married counterparts and have much lower levels of educational attainment. The same was true for the men they had children with. Even though the women were younger, they were more likely than their married counterparts to have children by another partner (McLanahan et al., 2010). In addition, the unwed mothers had much lower earnings than their married counterparts and were in poorer health and either used illegal drugs and or alcohol and were more likely to have partners that had a prison record. Finally, the study found that unwed couples were less likely to form stable unions. The majority of these couples experienced dissolution in their relationship 5 years after the birth of a child (McLanahan et al., 2010). The results from this study indicate that the characteristics of unwed parents discussed above are associated with poor outcomes for children of these parents (McLanahan et al., 2010). In particular, test scores and behavior problems were closely associated with relationship instability. While these findings do not specifically reflect results for African American female-headed households, many of the characteristics the authors drew attention to are also found among women in the African American community who have children out of wedlock.

It should be noted that some researchers have observed that the effects of the single-female–headed family structure on African American children may actually be mitigated by the unique characteristics of the African American community and culture. In particular, Fomby and Cherlin (2007) have noted that the negative characteristics associated with female family headship do not necessarily produce negative outcomes in cognitive performance or behavior problems (Fomby & Cherlin, 2007). According to this line of research, African American children are more likely to have access to extended family members who may offset the potential negative effects of single-parenting.

The analysis of social problems associated with female-headed families has been well documented. The creation of these households has been linked to a number of issues that have remained unresolved in the African American community. In addition, once these households are formed, there are a host of problems associated with them, including but not limited to, issues of poverty and welfare dependency as well as compromised well-being outcomes for the children in these families. The next section of the paper will examine the policies that have been implemented in the United States to address the problems associated with single-female–headed households.

PUBLIC POLICY APPROACHES TO SINGLE-PARENT FAMILIES

Since much of the research and discussion of African American female-headed households has examined these households as a problem that warrants fixing, public policies and programs that target these families have focused on ways in which the problems associated with these families can be treated or the extent to which the prevalence of this particular type of family structure can be reduced. Subsequently, in the public policy arena, the historic approach to dealing with single-parent families has been to attempt to replace what is missing. The replacement of what is missing has largely been done from a patriarchal perspective. Thus, given the insufficient income many of these families experience, public policy has attempted to replace the income of the absent father through public assistance programs. When these programs came under scrutiny, public policy shifted to creating programs whereby the government would not replace the income of the absent father, but mothers would become breadwinners for their families. Thus, under welfare reform, policies and programs were created to establish women as both breadwinners and caretakers through programs that encouraged work and "self-sufficiency." In addition, when welfare reform ideas emerged, the promotion of marriage and the reduction of out-of-wedlock births were also introduced as policies to reduce single-female–headed families. What has largely been neglected is how the issues associated with these families can be addressed through a more ecological and universal approach to public policy.

Income Maintenance and Single-Parent Families

Providing mothers with income in the absence of a father in the home has a long history in the United States. Starting in the early 1900s, several states began implementing programs to assist single mothers with children through what has come to be known as the Mothers Pension Programs (Leff, 1973). The goal of these programs was to keep women in the home with children rather than place them in orphanages or send women out to work (Leff, 1973). Those promoting the Mothers Pension Programs in the states argued that women could not simultaneously be adequate caretakers of children and breadwinners (Vandepol, 1982). Initially, these programs in the stats were primarily limited to women with children who had become single because of the death of their husbands. However, in a few cases, states allowed women outside of this category (i.e., women who had husbands who were incapacitated in some way, were divorced, or were in prison) to take advantage of the programs (Leff, 1973). In addition, it was usually the case that minority women were excluded from the benefit. African American women received a very small percentage of all the Mothers Pensions funds, and in some states, the southern states in particular, were not allowed to participate in the program (Leff, 1973). Thus, the initial approach to helping single-female–headed households was to use the state to replace the income of a father/husband who was legitimately removed from the family. However, in doing so, the Mothers Pension Program also laid the foundation for excluding families from the program who had an unemployed or underemployed male in the household. The demand that such men be "removed" from the household in order for the family to receive aid is the cornerstone of later policies and practices that promoted women making a choice between receiving assistance and having a stable relationship with a significant other. The exclusion of minority women from the benefit was premised on the expectation that such women, even if their husbands had died, should work for the keep of their children and themselves.

In 1935, with the passage of the Social Security Act, the idea of assisting single mothers with children was implemented in all states. Aid to Dependent Children (ADC), Title IV of the Social Security Act, was designed to provide financial assistance to children in single-female–headed households. In 1962 Congress amended the Social Security Act to create Aid to Families with Dependent Children (AFDC; Abronowitz, 2006). Unlike its predecessor (ADC), AFDC was designed to provide support to not only the children in single-female–headed households but the head of the household as well, something that ADC did not take into consideration. Both ADC and AFDC in their approach to helping single mothers with children sought to offer income support to these families. Both programs were structured around the ideological premise that in the absence of a male bread winner in the household, the state would be used as a substitute bread winner.

From 1935 to the early 1980s, the idea of providing a substitute income to single-female–headed households seemed to be the main goal of the ADC/AFDC programs. Prior to the 1960s, many of the households that were headed by women in the United States were created as a consequence of widowhood or separation and or divorce for women who had been married. In addition, prior to the 1960s, African American women were not disproportionately represented among women receiving benefits from the AFDC program. After 1960s, the population receiving AFDC had drastically changed. Women with children who had never been married and minority women began to crowd the AFDC rolls. Some of the criticisms of the AFDC program that had existed for some time began to gain a great deal more momentum as the country entered the 1980s. It was during this period that some in policy circles began to make the argument that the program encouraged out-of-wedlock births, discouraged marriage, and created long-term dependency on welfare rather than work as a means of support.

Criticisms of AFDC

Many of the criticisms aimed at the AFDC program were created using African American single-female–headed households as the example of what was wrong with welfare policy in the United States. The image of African American women and children has long been linked to welfare in a negative way (Quadango, 1984), but since these families were undoubtedly disproportionately represented among female-headed households in the United States, it became much easier to use them as the example of why welfare needed to be reformed. Based on the popular image of the African American single female on AFDC, criticisms of welfare were multifaceted, but two issues seemed to preoccupy those who called for the reformation of welfare. The first issue was the perceived length of time women spent on welfare (namely AFDC) and the number of children women birthed while receiving AFDC.

The first criticism of AFDC centered on the argument that the program encouraged long-term dependency rather than self-sufficiency through work (Downing, 2011). Critics argued that AFDC programs provided little or no incentive for women to seek education and/or job training to enter the labor market. Consequently, AFDC was perceived by some as a program that promoted long-term welfare dependency in women because they never acquired additional education or skills. This issue of dependency was coupled with the issue of poverty. Since AFDC did not provide support that lifted families out of poverty, the idea that continuing the program as is created and maintained a population of poor women and children also became an issue. This criticism was strongly promoted despite findings that women who become chronically dependent on AFDC were actually a small minority of AFDC recipients (McLanahan, 1988; McLanahan & Garfinkel, 1989). Thus, the notion that long-term dependency among single-female–headed households on AFDC created a large army of the underclass was actually a myth. It is actually the case that women are likely to stay on welfare in spells, rather than for chronically long periods of time (Harris, 1993).

The second criticism was one of the more controversial ones and has a long record of debate. Critics of AFDC also argued the program encouraged an increase in out-of-wedlock births in the African American community. The program did this in two ways according to critics. First, since women received additional cash assistance for each additional child they had, some argued that AFDC encouraged women to have additional children knowing that AFDC would provide support to these children. Second, some questioned whether the program actually discouraged marriage by making it more difficult for couples rather than single women to qualify for the benefit. The criticisms of AFDC as it related to African American women created momentum to reform the program. Proponents of the reform argued that public assistance for women should provide a hand-up rather than a handout. With that in mind, the dismantling of the AFDC program began.

Welfare Reform and Single-Parent Families

The overhauling of the AFDC program was heavily guided by the criticisms outlined above. However, in addition to these criticisms, there was the perception by many that AFDC was being used primarily by African American women. The perception of African American women as welfare queens was an entrenched image associated with AFDC despite the reality that the majority of women receiving the benefit were actually Caucasian women (Crass, 1998). The idea that African American women and not Caucasian women were utilizing the AFDC program was a major departure from the population policy makers had in mind when the Mothers Pension, ADC, and AFDC programs were originally implemented. The image of White women who had been widowed was the ideal recipient of these programs rather than Black women who were never married and had children out of wedlock. The perceived growth of the latter population on the AFDC rolls troubled policy makers.

In 1996, Congress passed the Personal Responsibility Work Opportunity Reconciliation Act. This piece of legislation has become synonymous with welfare reform. The legislation overhauled the AFDC program and created TANF. With African American mothers in mind, policy makers sought to restructure how single women with children were supported in the United States. There were several central policies implemented under welfare reform that seemed to address the perception of African American women receiving "too much" welfare support for too long. First, welfare support would become a temporary form of assistance tied to work. Single mothers with children would be required to find and maintain employment with the expectation of self-sufficiency. Second, no additional support would be provided for mothers who birthed additional children while on welfare. Third, states could compete for bonus money to reduce their out-of-wedlock birth rates, and fourth, the promotion of marriage was viewed as a policy that could be implemented to reduce reliance on welfare.

Temporary Assistance to Needy Families and Work

One of the primary goals of welfare reform was to get single mothers with children off of welfare and into the work force. Some research has indicated that for African American mothers on welfare, this was a much more difficult task compared to their White counterparts (Downing, 2011; Gooden, 1998). African American mothers were less likely to receive assistance from caseworkers in welfare agencies in finding work. Case managers were much more likely to assist White welfare recipients rather than African American recipients (Downing, 2011; Gooden, 1998). Research has also indicated that once African American women found employment, they earned lower wages compared to their White counterparts. Thus, White women were more likely to exit welfare into employment compared to their African American counterparts (Harris, 1993). Harris suggests that the more timely exit of White women from welfare into work and their higher wages compared to their African American counterparts may be due to the human capital advantage White women have over African American women (Harris, 1993).

The work policy instituted under welfare reform, which was designed to move African American women into the roles of breadwinner and caretaker, is inherently flawed. Given the difficulty African American women experience transitioning off of welfare in addition to the low wages that are earned by this population, they find themselves in a double bind—unable to fulfill either role particularly well. Women who transition off of welfare into low-paying jobs often find it difficult to arrange and pay for adequate child care. In addition, the low wages associated with the employment they find make it difficult to adequately provide the basic life necessities to their children.

Child Exclusion Policy and Illegitimacy Reduction Grants

The child exclusion policy implemented under welfare reform as well as the grant incentives given to states to reduce out-of-wedlock births were also designed with African American women in mind. Again, the perception of an out-of-control out-of-wedlock birth population in the African American community prompted discussions on how to handle the issue.

One of the beliefs popularized by Charles Murray in his book *Losing Ground* (1984) was that liberal welfare programs like AFDC promoted out-of-wedlock births. The argument popularized by Murray was that additional benefits paid to women who had additional children somehow incentivized having additional children (Murray, 1984). This was an argument conservatives picked up on and ran with in their promotion of the child exclusion policy under welfare reform. They believed cutting additional children from benefits would discourage women from having additional children. In addition to the child exclusion policy, states were encouraged to come up with ways to reduce their out-of-wedlock birth or illegitimacy rates. The five states that experienced the largest drop in their rate of out-of-wedlock births would each receive a $20 million bonus (Abronowitz, 2006).

The Child Exclusion and Illegitimacy Reduction Grants were ultimately designed to send the message that African American women who stepped outside the legitimate patriarchal definition of family (married with children) were not acceptable, and the state would no longer be responsible for children born into these households. Welfare reform reinforced the message that if you were going to have children outside of legitimate means, then as a woman, you should be prepared to work to take care of those children and be the primary caretaker of those children as well. Welfare reform essentially amounted to the abdication of state financial responsibility for single-female–headed households. Since African American women were disproportionately represented in this population, the policies of welfare reform had a powerful impact on this community.

Marriage Initiatives

The 1996 PRWORA included language that sought to promote marriage as a means of ending dependency on welfare (Fineman, Mink, & Smith, 2003). However, it was not until 2002, when PRWORA came up for reauthorization, that the Bush administration proposed funding states to promote marriage to the general public through advertising pro-marriage classes and divorce-avoidance classes for TANF recipients (Fineman et al., 2003). In February of 2003, the welfare reform reauthorization bill was passed. The bill included $500 million over a 5-year period for states to promote marriage not only to the general population but to TANF recipients in particular (Fineman et al., 2003). The popular wisdom was that if marriage made a difference in the economic and social well-being of families that were middle class and upper class, then surely marriage would do the same for lower-income individuals. In addition, specific promotion of marriage programs was created for specific populations. The African American Promotion of Marriage Institute specifically targets African Americans for the promotion of marriage goals.

The promotion of marriage as a response to poverty among single women who are heads of household provides us with an example of how far the devolution of responsibility for the poor (especially African American single women with children) has evolved. Welfare reform has not only given far more responsibility to states rather than the federal government to take care of these families, but the Promotion of Marriage Programs provides an example of further devolution of responsibility from the state to the private realm (Fineman et al., 2003; Cohen, 2010). The Promotion of Marriage places the responsibility for poor families on what policy makers see as the ideal family form: a two-parent heterosexual family in which one (preferably the husband) and/or both parents work. The attempt to move the care of single African American poor women with children to the realm of marriage for support is the ultimate abdication of state responsibility for this population. This agenda has drawn some positive responses among those who see the increase in African American female-headed household, the decrease in marriage among African Americans, and the increase in divorce and separation rates as destabilizing forces in the African American community. Proponents of this view see African American female-headed households as problematic, not only because they defy the accepted mainstream patriarchal notion of family but also because these families are associated with issues such as poverty, welfare reliance, and compromised child social well-being outcomes.

A salient criticism of this perspective and the marriage initiative in general is related to who these women being targeted for this intervention will marry. According to research mentioned previously, the male marriage pool for the population that is targeted by this intervention is limited because of a number of issues, including but not limited to unemployment, limited education, poor health, mortality, and incarceration. These issues have only been tangentially addressed by Marriage Initiative Programs through what is sometimes referred to as Fatherhood Initiative Programs. One of the major problems with welfare reform with respect to promoting self-sufficiency and marriage is that welfare reform programs have done very little to help move African American men who need help to economic self-sufficiency so that they can support or help support their families. According to Cohen (2010), of the $150 million that is allocated by the Department of Health and Human Services for the Healthy Marriage Initiative program, only $50 million is used to promote education and training of fathers through various Fatherhood Initiative Programs.

As discussed previously, the disproportionate percentage of single-female–headed households in the African American community is tied to systemic issues that limit the availability of men who are considered marriage partners for women. Two of the most salient issues in the African American community that have contributed to disparate rates of single-parenthood because of non marriage are the financial and educational disparities between African American men and women (Cohen, 2010). In addition, when examining the population that is being targeted for marriage promotion—poor women with children—the ability to find a mate who has the educational and income capacity to care for a family becomes even more limited. It should also be noted that the women that the Health Marriage Initiative targets are women who themselves have limited educational attainment and job skills that will allow them to find employment that would provide wages to help support a family. It is unlikely that the population the Healthy Marriage Initiative targets would be able to provide for a family without two incomes. Thus, the educational attainment, job skills, and income of both the men and women who are targeted is important to consider. As mentioned previously, very few programs seek to redress the issues facing African American men that have limited their availability in the marriage pool. This is not a new way of treating African American men.

As a society, we have partially placed the blame for increase in single-female–headed households in the African American community on women. Arguments supporting how or why women have contributed to this increase have been varied. One explanation is that African American women's attitudes toward marriage and out-of-wedlock childbearing have changed in order to accommodate the limited availability of men. In addition, prior to welfare reform, conservatives pushed the argument that African American women, even if they had a significant other in their lives, preferred to remain single in order to continue receiving benefits from AFDC. With respect to African American men, we have also placed blame on them for the increase in single-female–headed families in the African American community. After slavery in the United States, we expected African American men to take on the private patriarchal role as husband, father, and provider. The expectation was that African American families must provide for themselves rather than the state or federal government. This expectation was upheld even in the face of a history of discriminatory practices that prevented many African American men from accessing the resources that would allow them to adequately support families. Even after anti-discriminatory legislation, African American men found themselves competing in a labor market that had changed dramatically since the manufacturing heyday. While African American men may have been able to find employment to support a family during the 1950s and 1960s, the picture has shifted dramatically. The old manufacturing and production jobs that were once located in many of the inner cities populated by high concentrations of African Americans have dwindled (Wilson, 1996).

Instead, these jobs have given way to the availability of service industry jobs, which for persons with limited educational attainment translate into low wages.

At the same time, access to welfare programs that would allow African American men to support families has been very limited. For example, when the Social Security Act was passed in 1935, agricultural and domestic workers were excluded from the Old Age Insurance and Unemployment Insurance Programs (Davies & Derthick, 1997; Quadagno, 1984). The exclusion of these workers meant that a large portion of the African American population was excluded from these programs. White men and their families, on the other hand, were allowed to reap the benefits of federal government support. As our welfare state continued to develop, it has primarily focused on establishing ways to create breadwinners and caretakers out of African American women and has, for the most part, continued to ignore the plight of African American men. The expectation created under welfare reform, that African American men will become responsible for the care of their families through marriage, will require a broad-based approach that has not yet been an integral part of our welfare state. A discussion of what such an approach would entail is discussed below.

AN ECOLOGICAL-UNIVERSAL-COMMUNITY-BASED APPROACH TO THE ISSUE OF SINGLE-PARENT, FEMALE-HEADED HOUSEHOLDS IN THE AFRICAN AMERICAN COMMUNITY

Public policies that have attempted to address the issue of female-headed households have focused on three areas that all seek to solidify patriarchal expectations of families in our society. These areas include the replacement of absent fathers through income maintenance programs; the making of mothers into both caretaker and breadwinner through the implementation of welfare reform; and under welfare reform, an emphasis on marriage initiatives. To date, there is little evidence that any of these approaches has worked well in addressing the problems associated with these families.

Historically, public assistance programs such as ADC and AFDC, which were designed to use the state as a means of replacing income of a male head of household, created a set of other social problems. For example, ADC and AFDC, through rules and practices, encouraged women to stay single rather than marry. In addition, given the amount of assistance these programs provided to women and the limited training and education provided to women on the program, some argued the programs maintained women in poverty and fostered dependency rather than lifting women out of poverty. While welfare reform efforts during the 1980s and 1990s sought to redress the issues of dependency and poverty by promoting self-sufficiency through work, welfare reform initiatives have done very little to address the systemic issues that continue to keep women with children in poverty despite their exit from welfare and entrance into the labor force. Women who have exited welfare as a consequence of welfare reform still find themselves living under a cloud of income, food, housing, and health care insecurity. Finally, the emphasis that has been placed on the Healthy Marriage Initiative under welfare reform attempts to privatize the responsibility of care for poor single women with children. This effort can be interpreted as an extreme form of the devolution that has occurred with respect to the care of the poor in the United States, particularly poor African American women with children. While the idea of promoting marriage and subsequently strengthening what have been referred to as fragile families is an admirable endeavor, the initiative has included very few initiatives that would address the issues that prevent African American men and women from entering into stable marriages in the first place.

It is interesting to note that the public policy treatment of African American single-parent families has been largely framed from a patriarchal perspective. Policies have generally attempted to replace and/or supplement what is considered the missing link in these families: a male spouse who is a breadwinner. Sometimes, policies have emphasized one role more so than the other. For example, under welfare reform, more emphasis was placed on the breadwinner role of women rather than the integration of men into these families. The public policies that have tried to address the issue of single-parenting in the African American community have primarily implemented treatments that do not take into consideration the larger systemic issues that have contributed to the formation of these families. In addition, public policies to date have focused on treating these families in isolation from their ecological context. We propose that public policies that truly seek to address the issue of single-parenting in the African American community must at a minimum incorporate two features. First, programs and policies must take an ecological approach to treating these families. Second, policies and programs must emphasize providing access to resources that do not just reach single-parent families but emphasize the strengthening of all families. This requires the implementation of what is commonly referred to as universal programs.

PUBLIC POLICIES AND PROGRAMS: INCORPORATING AN ECOLOGICAL PERSPECTIVE

The ecological perspective or model of behavior proposed by Bronfenbrenner (1977) provides a useful tool for developing policies and programs that address the issue of single-female–headed families in the African American community. According to Bronfenbrenner, there are various levels of environmental influence on human behavior and interaction. These include the micro-system, meso-system, and exo-system. The micro-system refers to the day-to-day face-to-face interactions that shape and influence behaviors. The meso-system can best be described as the interconnections between the institutions in which individuals are embedded; for example, within communities, schools, churches, peer groups, and places of employment. Finally, the exo-system refers to the larger macro-forces in society in which families are embedded. These would include cultural beliefs, the economy, and the polity.

Examining single-female–headed families from an ecological perspective requires examining the social environmental factors that contribute to the creation of these families, the problems these families experience, and possible solutions to the problems associated with these families. As discussed previously, one of the most salient factors that has been identified in contributing to the increase in single-female–headed households in the African American community is the plight of African American men with respect to the factors that may prevent them from entering into stable marriage relationships. If one of the goals of public policy is to create stable families through marriage, then as practitioners we must advocate for the implementation of policies and programs that promote access to education, training, employment, and health and mental health services for African American men.

While the welfare state has historically developed programs to assist White men and White women and, reluctantly, minority women, programs that specifically address the issues facing African American men have not been a priority in the welfare state. If one of the goals of addressing the problems associated with single-female–headed households is to reduce the prevalence of these households through marriage, then the welfare state will have to incorporate programs that specifically meet the needs of African American men. Based on the complexity of factors that have contributed to the increase in single-female–headed households in the African American community, there is very little evidence that the growth of single-female–headed families can be reversed in a short period of time. Given this reality, a question we should address is how an ecological perspective can assist us in developing policies and programs to strengthen these families.

A Universal Approach to Public Policies and Programs

Policy Practice

To date, the majority of programs that have attempted to address the needs of African American single-parent female-headed families have been means-tested programs. Programs such as ADC, AFDC, TANF, Medicaid, and Food Stamps (now SNAP) are designed to treat the poor, and in the public's mind, are perceived as programs that are overwhelmingly populated by African American female-headed families. These programs have been highly stigmatized in American society because of the population the programs are designed to serve. Such programs, over time, have isolated the poor and until recently encouraged separation from the labor market (McLanahan & Garfinkel, 1989). The idea that poor African American women with children received "special treatment" and did not have to work but could be supported by the state further stigmatized this population in the public's mind. Subsequently, programs that seek to treat these families have been designed to punish a population that is viewed as living outside of the bounds of societal expectations concerning family, childbearing, and work. As a consequence, these programs have been designed to offer these families a subsistence level of support rather than lifting these families out of poverty and into self-sufficiency.

Universal programs would provide assistance to all families in need irrespective of income level. Such programs are capable of helping families out of poverty without stigmatizing them. This is so because programs that are universal tend to garner greater support from mainstream society because they are potentially designed to reach all families. As a consequence, these programs tend to be funded much more liberally compared to categorical means-tested programs (McLanahan & Garfinkel, 1989; Wilson, 1987).

Based on the problems associated with single-female–headed families explored in this paper, it is clear that public policies that are designed to help families must emphasize lifting families out of poverty and sustaining them by providing them with those life necessities that all families require to thrive. Many African American single-female–headed families require resources that would be advantageous to all families irrespective of their family structure or incomes. In our society, no family is truly self-sufficient. All families require access to resources that will assist them with their well-being. It is clear that despite the recent emphasis on marriage for single-parent families, increasing marriage in and of itself may not be the solution to the issue of single-parenting in the African American community. Some researchers have even questioned whether we need to continue to frame these families from a deficit perspective rather than a strengths perspective. These researchers ask the question, If we can't or shouldn't engineer marriage through policies and programs, what supports do African American single-parent families need in order to thrive?

We contend that ensuring some of the most basic necessities have been half-heartedly addressed by welfare policies in the United States. First and foremost, one of the most salient issues facing families, but in particular African American single-parent families, is the ability to earn an income that is considered a living wage. If we expect families to be self-sufficient through employment, we must promote policies that make a serious commitment to providing education and training to women and men that prepare them for jobs that pay a living wage. In addition to adequate income, affordable and convenient child care and affordable housing are still issues that have not been resolved for families in the United States. If we expect heads of families to work to support themselves, we must also be willing to assist families with acquiring affordable child care and housing. Work becomes less attractive when families have to spend a large portion of their incomes on child care. In addition, the increasing limited availability of low- and moderate-priced housing in the United States means that families are spending a significant portion of the incomes they earn on shelter. All families could benefit from programs that focus on promoting access to these three life necessities.

However, we must also be prepared to recognize that for various reasons, heads of families will be separated from the labor market for periods of time. The present recession is a good example of one such time. Given this inevitability, we must promote policies that provide income and in-kind supports that mitigate the negative outcomes associated with poverty.

The Role of Direct Practice at the Community Level

Apart from policies and programs that need to be implemented on the federal level, we also need to consider the role of communities in shaping outcomes for families. Strong communities are those in which access to quality education, health care, affordable housing, civic organizations, recreational outlets, and employment are readily accessible. Families that live in communities that experience deficits in these resources are at risk for many of the problems previously discussed. In today's society, African American single-female heads of household are more likely to find themselves isolated in communities with deficits in these resources. This makes it difficult not only for them to escape poverty and become self-sufficient but also provide their children with those things they need to experience optimal well-being. In addition, communities with deficits in these areas make it difficult for these women to find acceptable marriage partners. As practitioners, we also need to consider the resources that are lacking in communities and the ways in which these resources can be introduced into communities.

In addition to strengthening community resources, we argue that the notion of strengthening couples and marriage should also be examined as a direct practice intervention. There is evidence that despite the decline in marriage and increase in female-headed households, African Americans value marriage. The value of marriage in the African American community along with the strong ties of African Americans to the faith-based community are strengths that can be used to build programs that promote stability in couple relationships and marriage. In particular, the church can be used as a resource to offer a variety of programs that promote healthy personal development in young men and women, provide education on marriage, and offer supports to married couples. Such programs could also be offered through nonprofit voluntary organizations.

Programs that focus on healthy personal development in young men and women should provide young people with assistance in successfully completing education and training, sex education, and communication and conflict resolution skills. Marriage education programs would focus on providing information about the benefits of marriage for men and women as well as children. While there are programs that are in existence that are designed to help couples in trouble, many of these programs do not take into account the unique cultural and structural issues African American couples experience. The implementation of these programs in African American communities will have to take these factors into account.

Research Implications

While we now have a relatively clear understanding of the factors that have produced the increase in female-headed households and the decline in marriage in the African American community, it is relatively clear what types of policies and programs need to be implanted that address the economic and social welfare issues that have led to the increase in female-headed households. What is less clear is how this issue can be addressed through the use of marriage-promotion programs in direct practice. While marriage programs have a relatively long history in the United States, many of these programs are not necessarily culturally competent with respect to taking into account the unique cultural and structural experiences of African Americans. Research is needed to determine which models and practices associated with marriage programs are best suited for promoting and maintaining marriage in the African American community. In particular, given the strength of the church in the African American community, research is also needed to determine the types of ministries, services, and programs churches have already engaged in and the effectiveness of these.

REFERENCES

Abronowitz, M. (2006). Welfare reform in the United States: Gender, race and class matter. *Critical Social Policy, 26*(2), 336–364.

Akerlof, G., Yellen, J., & Katz, M. (1996). An analysis of out of wedlock childbearing in the United States. *The Quarterly Journal of Economics, 11*(2), 277–317.

Baker, D. (1999). The increase of single-parent families: An examination of causes. *Policy Sciences, 32*, 175–188.

Billingsley, A. (1968). *Black families in white America*. Englewood Cliffs, NJ: Prentice-Hall.

Billingsley, A. (1992). *Climbing Jacob's Ladder: The enduring legacy of African American families*. New York: Simon and Schuster.

Brodsky, A. (1999). Making it: The components and process of resilience among urban, African American, single mothers. *American Journal of Orthopsychiatry, 69*(2), 148–160.

Bronfenbrenner, U. (1977). Toward an experimental ecology of human development. *American Psychologist, 32*(7), 513–531.

Carlson, M., Garfinkel, I., McLanahan, S., Mincy, R., & Primus, W. (2004). The effects of welfare and child support policies on union formation. *Population Research and Policy Review, 23*, 513–542.

Chaney, C. (2011). The Character Of Womanhood: How African American women's perceptions of womanhood influence marriage and motherhood. *Ethnicities, 11*(4), 512–535.

Cohen, R. (2010). Two steps forward, one step back: Evaluating the Healthy Marriage Initiative in light of America's welfare history. *Georgetown Journal on Poverty Law and Policy, 17*, 145–157.

Crass, C. (2004). Beyond welfare queens: Developing a race, class and gender analysis of welfare and welfare reform. *Colors of Resistance, 3*.

Davies, G., & Derthick, M. (1997). Race and social welfare policy: The Social Security Act of 1935. *Political Science Quarterly, 112*(2), 217–235

DeNavas,-Walt, C., Proctor, B. D., & Smith, J. C. (2011). *Income, poverty and health insurance coverage in the United States: 2010 U.S. Census Bureau, Current Population Reports*. (pp. 60–239). Washington, DC: U.S. Government Printing Office.

Dickson, L. The future of marriage and family in black America. (1993). *Journal of Black Studies, 23*(4), 472–491.

Dominguez, S., and Watkins, C. (2003). Creating networks for survival and mobility: Social capital among African American and Latin American low-income mothers. *Social Problems, 50*(1), 111–135.

Downing, K. (2011). A literature review of the experiences of African American and Caucasian TANF women transitioning from welfare to work. *Journal of Human Behavior in the Social Environment, 21*, 25–34.

Fineman, M., Mink, G., & Smith, M. (2003). No promotion of marriage in TANF. *Social Justice, 30*(4), 126–134.

Fomby, P., & Cherlin, A. (2007). Family instability and child well being. *American Sociological Review, 72*, 181–204.

Foster, H. (1983). African patterns in the Afro-American Family. *Journal of Black Studies, 14*(2), 201–232.

Gooden, S. (1998) All things not being equal: Difference in caseworker support toward black and white clients. *Harvard Journal of African American Public Policy, 4*, 23–33.

Goodwin, P. (2003). African American and European American women's marital well-being. *Journal of Marriage and Family, 65*, 550–560.

Harknet, K., & Hartnett, C. (2011). Who lacks support and why? An explanation of mothers' personal safety nets. *Journal of Marriage and Family, 73*, 861–875.

Harris, K. (1993). Work and welfare among single mothers in poverty. *American Journal of Sociology, 99*(2), 317–352.

Hill, R. The strengths of black families (2nd ed.). Oxford, UK: University Press of America 2003.

Holzer, H. (2009). The labor market and young black men: Updating Moynihan's perspective. *Annals of the American Academy of Political Science, 621*, 47–69.

Irving, S. K. (2011). *Comparing program participation of TANF and non TANF families before and during time of recession. Current Population Reports* (pp. 70–127). Washington, DC: U.S. Census Bureau.

Jayakody, R., & Kalil, A. (2002). Social fathering in low income, African American families with preschool children. *Journal of Marriage and Family. 64*(2), 504–516.

King, A. E. O. (1999). African American females' attitudes toward marriage: An exploratory study. *Journal of Black Studies, 29*(3), 416–437.

Leff, M. H. (1973). Consensus for reform: The Mothers' Pension Movement in the progressive era. *Social Service Review, 47*(3), 397–417.

Littlejohn-Blake, S. M., & Darling, C. Understanding the strengths of African American families. *Journal of Black Studies*, *23*(4) 460–471.

Lopoo, L., & Western, B. (2005). Incarceration and formation and stability of marital unions. *Journal of Marriage and Family*, *67*(3), 721–734.

McCreary, L., & Dancy, B. (2004). Dimensions of family functioning: Perspectives of low-income African American single-parent families. *Journal of Marriage and Family*, *66*(3), 690–701.

McLanahan, S. (1988). Family structure and dependency: Early transitions to female headed household headship. *Demography*, *25*, 1–16.

McLanahan, S., & Garfinkel, I. (1989). Single mothers, the underclass and social policy. *Annals of the American Academy of Political and Social Science*, *501*, 92–104.

McLanahan, S., Haskins, R., Garfinkel, I., Mincy, R., & Donahue, E. (2010). Strengthening fragile families. the future of children. Brookings Institute Policy Brief. Retrieved from www.brookings.edu

Moynihan, D. P. (1965). *The Negro family: The case for national action*. Washington, DC: U.S. Government Printing Office.

Murray, C. (1984). *Losing ground: American social policy 1950–1984*. New York, NY: Basic Books.

Persuad, N., Gray, P., & Hunt, E. (1999). Raised by African-American single-parents to succeed: The perspectives of children. *International Journals*, *29*(1), 69–84.

Pettit, B., & Western, B. (2004). Mass imprisonment and the life course: Race and class inequality in U.S. incarceration. *American Sociological Review*, *69*, 151–169.

Pinderhughes, E. (2002). African American marriage in the 20th century. *Family Process*, *41*(2), 269–282

Quadagno, J. S. (1984). Welfare capitalism and the Social Security Act of 1935. *American Sociological Review*, *49*(5), 632–647.

Rich, J. (2000). The health of African American men. *The Annals of the American Academy of Political and Social Science*, *569*, 149–159.

Ricketts, E. (1989). The origin of the black female headed families. *Focus, 12*(1), 32–36.

Roberts, D. (2004). The social and moral cost of mass incarceration in African American communities. *Stanford Law Review*, *56*(5), 1271–1305.

Rolison, G. (1992). Black, single female-headed family formation in large U.S. cities. *The Sociological Quarterly*, *33*(3), 473–481.

Staples, R. (1985). Changes in black family structure: The conflict between family ideology and structural conditions. *Journal of Marriage and the Family*, *47*, 1005–1015.

Travis, J. (2002). Invisible punishment: An instrument of social exclusion. In M. Mauer & M. Chesney-Lind (Eds.), *Invisible punishment: The collateral consequences of mass imprisonment* (pp. 15–36). New York: New Press.

Unnever, J. (2008). Two worlds far apart: Black-white differences in beliefs about why African-American men are disproportionately imprisoned. *Criminology*, *46*(2), 511–538.

Vandepol, A. (1982). Dependent children, child custody, and the Mothers' Pensions: The transformation of state-family relations in the early 20th century. *Social Problems*, *29*(3), 221–235.

Western, B., & Pettit, B. (2000). Incarceration and racial inequality in men's employment. *Industrial and Labor Relations Review*, *54*(1), 3–16/

Wilson, W. J. (1987). *The truly disadvantaged: The inner city, the underclass, and public policy*. Chicago, IL: University of Chicago Press.

Wilson, W. J. (1996). *When work disappears: The world of the new urban poor*. New York, NY: Alfred A. Knopf, Inc.

Index

Note: Page numbers in *italics* represent tables
Page numbers in **bold** represent figures